COLLABORATING WITH INTERPRETERS AND TRANSLATORS

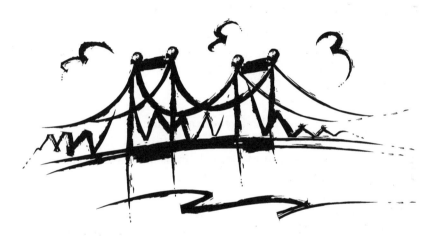

A Guide for
Communication Disorders Professionals

Henriette W. Langdon, EdD
Li-Rong Lilly Cheng, PhD

With a Foreword by Elisabeth H. Wiig, PhD

Thinking Publications • Eau Claire, Wisconsin

08 07 06 05 04 03 02 01   8 7 6 5 4 3 2 1

Library of Congress Catalog-in-Publication Data

Langdon, Henriette W., date.
    Collaborating with interpreters and translators: a guide for
    professionals in communication disorders / Henriette W. Langdon,
    Li-Rong Lilly Cheng.
        p. cm.
    Includes bibliographical references and index.
    ISBN 1-888222-76-X (pbk.)
      1. Speech therapy. 2. Audiology. 3. Translating and interpreting. I.
    Cheng, Li-Rong Lilly, date. II. Title.

    RC423 .L326 2002
    616.85'506—dc21   2001041469

Printed in the United States of America
Cover design by Kristin Kulig Sosalla

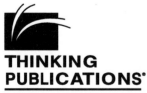

**THINKING
PUBLICATIONS®**

A Division of McKinley Companies, Inc.
424 Galloway Street • Eau Claire, WI 54703
(715) 832-2488 • FAX (715) 832-9082
Email: custserv@ThinkingPublications.com

COMMUNICATION SOLUTIONS THAT CHANGE LIVES®

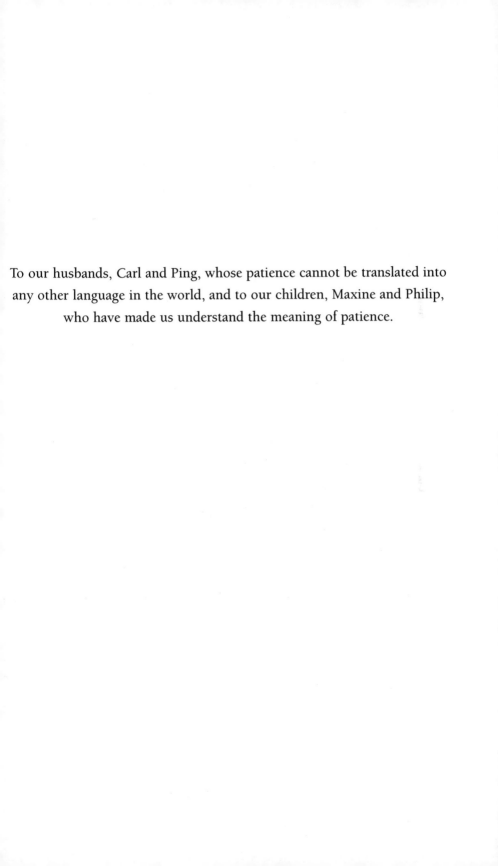

To our husbands, Carl and Ping, whose patience cannot be translated into any other language in the world, and to our children, Maxine and Philip, who have made us understand the meaning of patience.

ABOUT THE AUTHORS

Henriette W. Langdon, EdD, CCC-SLP, is an associate professor at San José State University in the Communicative Disorders and Sciences Department and is a fellow of the American Speech-Language-Hearing Association (ASHA). Henriette has more than 25 years of experience working with bilingual students who have a variety of speech, language, and learning disabilities. She has published several papers, book chapters, and books and has presented on this topic at state, national, and international levels. As a speaker of four different languages, one of her interests is the process of interpreting and translating and its relationship to practice in the fields of speech-language pathology and audiology.

Li-Rong Lilly Cheng, PhD, CCC-SLP, is a professor in the Department of Communicative Disorders at San Diego State University. Lilly has 30 years of experience working with bilingual children and adults. She has published several books and numerous professional articles. In addition, she has presented at state, national, and international levels. She is on the editorial board of several major journals and is a fellow of the American Speech-Language-Hearing Association (ASHA).

CONTENTS

LIST OF FIGURES AND TABLES

Figures

Tables

FOREWORD

This text should become standard fare for speech-language pathologists, clinical audiologists, translators, and interpreters who are collaborators in the process of creating meaning and understanding the difficult subjects and emotional issues we face in the communication disorders field. The text covers a broad range of topics and issues and presents excellent examples to support the discussions. The authors give readers insights into the challenges associated with mediating understanding between communication disorders professionals who communicate in American English and consumers who represent the diversity of languages and cultures of the globe. They provide structured models for process-oriented collaborative assessments and for training professionals to collaborate in a dynamic assessment and intervention process. The authors also speak eloquently on the roles and challenges associated with the collaborative efforts between communication disorders professionals and translators or interpreters. This is indeed a text that opens the mind to cultural and linguistic diversity and the challenges associated with it.

Many professionals who will gravitate toward this text, whether clinicians, interpreters, or translators, have experienced the culture shock that results when one either travels to or moves to a foreign country. Americans often travel on organized tours in countries where English is not the primary language. They are cushioned against, but not completely spared, the shocks of a foreign culture and language. Those who have traveled alone in a foreign country or immigrated to the United

States from non-English speaking societies know how difficult it can be to orient oneself culturally and linguistically and how lost one can feel in the new context.

Many years ago, I came to the United States from Scandinavia. I thought I could speak English and manage what America had to offer a foreign student immigrant. I was literate by both British and American standards, but I had not learned the everyday language and cultural conventions needed to function in real life. This was brought home to me in a very painful way when I needed surgery and could not explain where the pain was or understand what the nurses and doctors wanted me to do. There were no interpreters and no translators. Only one language could help us communicate: the language of universally functional gestures. The anxiety, sense of isolation, and sometimes panic I experienced prepared me to read this text and to appreciate what it has to offer.

This text can be read in many ways. You can read it as a professional with a general interest in the origins and comparative characteristics of the major languages of the world. You can read it to improve your understanding of the cultural and linguistic challenges so many people are faced with in the pursuit of the American dream. You can use the text as a reference work and read only what you need to know, when you need it. You can let yourself get into the totality of the text and gain a better understanding of the issues and methodologies involved in removing some of the barriers to cross-linguistic and cross-cultural communication. Finally, you can use the text for program planning and for educating professionals.

The voice of authenticity in the text comes from sources within the authors. Both are master clinicians and have contributed to the literature on bilingualism and cultural diversity in speech-language pathology and audiology. Both authors are immigrants to the United States and share the experience of culture shock with past and present immigrants. They complement each other because they share the challenges of the immigrant but they experienced different kinds of challenges in adapting to the American culture due to their differing origins—one Central European-Mexican, the other Chinese. In this text, the authors' personal voices come through loud and clear, yet in a scholarly way.

As mentioned earlier, this text is broad in scope and content. It features illustrative examples of points of potential conflict in the interpersonal communication between speakers of American English and consumers from different cultural/linguistic backgrounds. There are examples from, among others, Cantonese, Mandarin, Japanese, Vietnamese, German, Polish, and Spanish. The examples illustrate conflicts that can arise at the levels of content, form and use, and nonverbal communication. They underscore the multifaceted nature and dynamic interaction between these levels in different languages and cultures. There are also clinical cases that illustrate how the collaborative, process-oriented assessment model and its phases—briefing, interaction, and debriefing (BID)—play out in real life with speakers of Cambodian, Mandarin, Spanish, and Vietnamese. These case studies are in themselves invaluable. The text also includes excellent reference information on the origins, uses, and characteristics of the major language families and of individual languages of the world. The text is easy to read and provided me with new and exciting clinical models and information.

Elisabeth H. Wiig, PhD, CCC-SLP/A

PREFACE

Effective communication is achieved when individuals share the same linguistic, social, and cultural backgrounds because meanings are transmitted more readily and accurately. A greater challenge surfaces when two parties speak different languages. In these instances, the collaboration of an interpreter, for spoken communication, or translator, for written communication, is necessary to bridge the communication gap. As we have found through our own experiences as multilingual speakers, interpretation or translation goes beyond using equivalent words and expressions across two language systems. The process of interpretation or translation needs to consider the linguistic, cultural, and educational backgrounds of the people who are dependent on the interpreter in addition to the context in which the interaction is taking place. Therefore, being bilingual does not necessarily mean that one can be an effective interpreter or translator.

Today we have more information on interpretation in specific contexts, such as international conferences, court interpretation, interpretation services for the deaf, and, to some degree, medical interpretation. However, there is relatively little information on how to effectively collaborate with interpreters in an educational or clinical context. Knowledge of the field of interpretation is in its beginning stages because research in this field is very scant. However, with all nations, including the United States, experiencing an increasing number of speakers of various languages, it is necessary to understand and to explore the process of interpretation to maximize effective communication between individuals who do not share the same language.

Accurate translation is equally important when written information needs to be conveyed from one language to the other.

The purpose of this book is to provide a framework for responding to many of the challenges that occur when the services of an interpreter or translator are needed in the fields of speech-language pathology and audiology. The book includes six chapters and four appendices.

Chapter 1: Bridging Linguistic Diversity traces the history of interpreting and translating from their professional beginnings in the early 1920s following World War I and provides some general demographic language trends.

Chapter 2: Communicating in a Multilingual Society describes various language components such as dialect, phonology, semantics, and pragmatics. The role of code switching and language loss in a bilingual speaker's language use is defined. Normal and deviant patterns in code switching are described.

Chapter 3: Balancing Linguistic and Cultural Variables focuses on specific verbal, nonverbal, cultural, and contextual aspects of interpretation and translation. Answers are provided for many common questions that occur in the collaboration process.

Chapter 4: Assessing Culturally/Linguistically Diverse (CLD) Populations discusses the drawbacks of using standardized tests and the limited number of non-English tests. Suggestions are given for conducting assessments.

Chapter 5: Interpreting in Speech-Language Pathology and Audiology describes the roles and responsibilities of each one of the collaborative team members. It outlines the three-step process of briefing, interaction, and debriefing (BID) to be followed in interviews, conferences, assessments, and intervention.

Chapter 6: Enhancing Professional Development Programs and the Future of Interpreters outlines a suggested professional development program for interpreters working in speech-language pathology and audiology. Checklists are provided for evaluating members of the collaborative team. Activities to illuminate the future of interpreters are discussed.

Appendix A describes the top 10 most commonly spoken languages in the world.

Appendix B lists many speech-language and audiology tests in languages other than English.

Appendix C includes case studies that describe the collaboration of a speech-language pathologist and an interpreter working with three different clients: a 9-year-old Spanish speaker, a 5-year-old Mandarin speaker, and a 68-year-old Spanish speaker. A fourth collaboration is described between an audiologist and interpreter in the case of a 74-year-old Vietnamese speaker.

Appendix D presents a sample report where the speech-language pathologist used the services of an interpreter to assess a Cambodian-speaking preschool child.

ACKNOWLEDGMENTS

This book could not have become a reality without the support, encouragement, and effort of many people. First of all, I want to thank my friend, colleague, and coauthor Lilly Cheng. Having Lilly as coauthor of this book enabled both of us to be more thorough. Even though we can share only one language, English, combined we can communicate in more than seven languages. This is a minuscule accomplishment compared to the more than 6,000 different languages currently spoken on our planet. However, we hope that our readers will be able to gain a more complete perspective because the information has been filtered through more than one language. Thank you, Lilly.

Also, this book could not have been produced without the support of Nancy McKinley, editor in chief of Thinking Publications. Thank you, Nancy, for your interest in this topic, for your belief in our work, and for your willingness to help us create new pathways to solve a few of the many dilemmas facing us in our complex professions. The text became more clear and appealing because of the guidance, expertise, and excellent technical skills of our editors, Joyce Olson and Heather Johnson Schmitz. We thank you both for your hard work as you dedicated many hours and much thought to our book.

We would also like to thank Dr. Elisabeth Wiig for her willingness to offer very helpful suggestions on improving the quality of the book and for the thoughtful and supportive foreword she wrote.

We wish to thank the reviewers—Kathryn Kohnert, Mary Blake Huer, William Prather, and Elisabeth Wiig—who offered much constructive criticism.

Also, we thank Janna Lang and June McCullough for their frontline accounts of strategies they implement with their multicultural clients who need audiological services.

Finally, I would not have been able to be who I am without my parents' strong belief in multilingualism, multiculturalism, and understanding other people's thoughts and feelings, all of which has had a long-lasting effect in my personal and professional life.

Henriette W. Langdon, coauthor

1 Bridging Linguistic Diversity

Many voices, one song.
—Anonymous

Chapter Goals

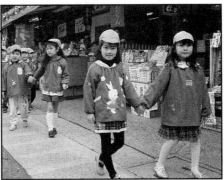

- Define the terms *interpretation* and *translation,* and offer a brief historical perspective of the process of interpreting and translating

- Identify the top 10 languages spoken in the world, language families, and the categories languages fall under

- Provide current and predicted demographic data on various linguistic groups living in the United States and their proficiency in English

- Discuss the need for interpreters and translators in the fields of speech-language pathology and audiology

- Explain the methods of interpreting and translating

DISCUSSION ITEMS

1. In what ways do you think the demand for interpreters and translators in the United States has changed between the early 1900s and today?

2. Why would it be important during a language assessment to know that the primary language of the client is an isolating language?

3. What are the most common languages spoken in your community? What sources of information can be used to find this information?

4. How might a speech-language pathologist or audiologist justify the need for an interpreter or translator?

5. What are some potential benefits and drawbacks of the two methods of interpreting?

HISTORICAL PERSPECTIVE OF INTERPRETERS AND TRANSLATORS

Interpretation and *translation* are complementary terms that may be used differentially depending on the context. For the purposes of this book, *interpretation* means conveying information from one language to another when the message is oral; *translation* means the message is written. In this book, the term *interpretation* will be used more often because it is the more common process. Although the differentiation of the two terms clarifies the process, it is sometimes difficult to separate interpreting from translating. In common usage, the two terms are often used interchangeably.

> [I]nterpretation means conveying information from one language to another when the message is oral; translation means the message is written.

Since ancient times, people who spoke different languages had to rely on the assistance of someone who could bridge the communication barrier. Prior to the twentieth century, translation was primarily used to convert the meaning of religious, literary, scientific, or philosophical texts (Baker and Jones, 1998). Likewise, the process of interpretation has been in existence for a long time, since two or more parties did not share the same spoken language. For example, when Cortez landed in the Americas in the 1500s, he had to rely on the assistance of someone who could communicate in both Spanish and the particular language spoken in the region. Similarly, Roberts (1997) reported that early French

3

settlers in Canada saw the need for interpreters and sent two native Iroquois speakers to France to be trained. However, upon their return to Canada, the interpreters never collaborated fully when there was a conflict of interests between the settlers and the natives. From that time on, a new trend reportedly began in which "French resident-interpreters adopted the Indian lifestyle and acted not only as linguistic intermediaries, but also as commercial agents, diplomats and guides" (Roberts, 1997, p. 7).

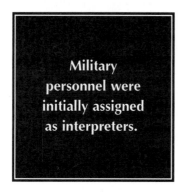

Military personnel were initially assigned as interpreters.

Until World War I, when two countries were at war, the official peace treaties were negotiated and written in French, no matter what the language of the warring countries was. It became apparent that French/English interpreters were needed by the United States during World War I peace negotiations. Military personnel were initially assigned as interpreters (Gerver and Sinaiko, 1977).

The increased participation of the United States in military affairs and the greater need for communication between various nations to enhance scientific and commercial exchanges were the basis for the creation of specific language-training centers. One of the first and most renowned centers was l'École d'Interprètes in Geneva, Switzerland, which offered training for interpreters who became available at various international conferences and the United Nations. Today, there are many schools that are famous worldwide, including the Monterey Institute in California and Georgetown University in Washington, DC.

With the advent of technology, the interpreter-training process may become more effective and widely accessible. Translations using computers are more accessible; however, a human element will always be needed to edit the information. Thus, trained bilingual and multilingual individuals will be in great demand to interpret and translate for all nations as these nations become increasingly multilingual and need to interact in a global society.

LANGUAGE DEMOGRAPHICS
Languages Spoken in the World

There are currently 6,500 identified languages in the world, though as many as 300 of these may be extinct (Nettle, 1999). The living languages are spoken in 200 countries. English, French, Spanish, or Arabic have been adopted as official languages in about 120 of these countries. As many as 45 other languages have regional recognition. However, only 1.5% of all languages have been accepted as international or have been recognized as "official languages." The rest, or 98.5%, have no official status (Baker and Jones, 1998).

There are languages that are spoken by millions of people and others that are spoken by only a few. In Africa alone, there are 222 languages, but many are facing extinction. In India, there are four language families and 37 languages, of which 5 are recently extinct, 6 are spoken by less than 20 speakers, 6 are shared by less than 100 speakers, and 14 are spoken by less than

500 speakers. More than 20 indigenous languages are spoken by less than 5,000 people in Canada. Almost 95% of the world's speakers use only 4% of the world's oral languages (Kallen, 2000). Of all the world's oral languages, 20 to 50% are no longer learned by children. By the year 2100, it is predicted that several hundred additional languages will be extinct (Fishman, 1991).

The number of primary and secondary speakers of a given language, the number of countries using the language, the number of major occupational fields communicating with the language, the economic power of the region where the language is spoken, and social prestige are all contributing factors in strengthening and preserving a given language (Baker and Jones, 1998). Chinese (Mandarin), Spanish, English, Bengali, Hindi, Portuguese, Russian, Japanese, German (Standard), and Chinese (Wu) are the top 10 languages of the world based on one or more of the factors listed above (Grimes, 1999). Information about various languages can be found in resources such as Baker and Jones (1998), Campbell (1995), Crystal (1997), and Katzner (1986). Table 1.1 lists the 10 major languages spoken in the world.

Table 1.2 (see page 8) lists the major language families in alphabetical order and includes examples. Familiarity with language names, origins, and general characteristics will help speech-language pathologists, audiologists, educators, resource teachers, school psychologists, and primary- and allied-health professionals understand more about the students and clients they encounter. Descriptions of the world's top 10 languages are included in Appendix A.

Challenges in translation and interpretation exist because

Table 1.1   **The World's Top 10 Spoken Languages**

Rank	Language	Primary Country	Number of Speakers
1	Chinese, Mandarin	China	885,000,000
2	Spanish	Spain	332,000,000
3	English	United Kingdom	322,000,000
4	Bengali	Bangladesh	189,000,000
5	Hindi	India	182,000,000
6	Portuguese	Portugal	170,000,000
7	Russian	Russia	170,000,000
8	Japanese	Japan	125,000,000
9	German, Standard	Germany	98,000,000
10	Chinese, Wu	China	77,175,000

Source: Grimes (1999)

of differences in the properties of languages and cultures. Among the 6,500 identified languages of the world, four main groups have been identified based on the importance of morphology in determining meaning (Comrie, 1992; Menn, O'Connor, Obler, and Holland, 1995). These four groups include (1) isolating (e.g., Chinese), (2) fusional or inflecting (e.g., German), (3) agglutinative (e.g., Japanese), and (4) polysynthetic (e.g., many Native American languages). *Isolating languages* are those where words are invariable and do not use inflections (e.g., prefixes and suffixes). In these languages, word order determines the meaning of what is said. In *fusional* or *inflecting languages*, word inflections add meaning to what is said. *Agglutinative languages* use combinations of inflections to

7

Table 1.2 **Major Language Families**

Language Families	Examples
Altaic	Japanese, Korean
Austro-Asiatic	Khmer, Vietnamese, Hmong
Germanic	English, German, Dutch, Scandinavian
Indic	Bengali, Hindu
Malayo-Polynesian	Tagalog, Chamorro
Romance	French, Spanish, Italian, Portuguese, Romanian
Slavic	Russian, Polish, Yugoslavian, and specific dialects such as Estonian, and Latvian
Sino-Tibetan	Mandarin, Thai, Lao, Cantonese

Source: Cheng (1995)

a word to denote different categories, such as person, number, tense, voice, and mood. P*olysynthetic languages*, not among the most commonly spoken, combine individual word elements into a composite word that would be expressed as a phrase or sentence in most other languages.

Today, more than ever before, many countries with a majority language, such as French or German, report a greater diversity of languages spoken among their residents because of immigration. For example, languages that are spoken in Germany include Italian, Spanish, Greek, Turkish, Portuguese, and Yugoslavian. Some countries include one or more official languages and several other languages and dialects. For example, in Ethiopia there are 15 regional languages, 50 to 70 different regional varieties, and two official languages (Oromo and Amharic). Australia includes speakers of English and a large population of speakers of Italian, Greek, various dialects of Chinese and Arabic, German, Vietnamese, and Spanish. Seventy-five different languages are spoken in Ghana, and most of the population, estimated to be about 18 million, speaks two or more languages (Baker and Jones, 1998).

An understanding of the complexities of the various languages is imperative to achieve successful oral and written communication between individuals who do not share the same language. Therefore, communication disorders professionals need to understand the levels of proficiency of the interpreter or translator with whom they work and the many complex factors and challenges they face. See Chapter 3 for more information on these topics.

Languages Spoken in the United States

Figure 1.1 (see page 10) compares the main population groups living in the United States in 1995 with trends predicted for 2050. The White (Caucasian) population will decrease from 73.5% to 51.2% of the total population, whereas the Hispanic and Asian and Pacific Islander population will increase two-fold and three-fold respectively.

Fourteen percent of the United States population ages 5 years and over, or 31.8 million people, speak a language other than English at home. Spanish is the language most frequently spoken (about 54%). Between 1980 and 1990, a decline in the number

Population Change between 1995 and 2050 in the United States

Figure 1.1

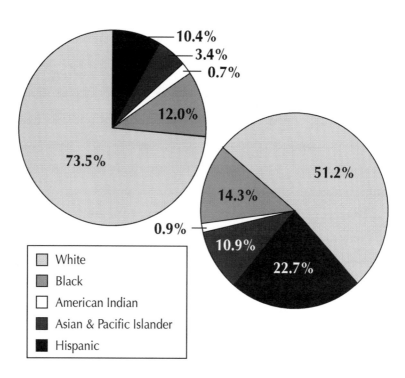

From *Encyclopedia of Bilingualism and Bilingual Education* (p.447), by C. Baker and S.P. Jones, 1998, Clevedon, England: Multilingual Matters. © 1998 by Multilingual Matters. Reprinted with permission.

of speakers of Italian, Polish, Greek, and German in the United States was reported; however, during that same period, the number of speakers of Vietnamese, Hindi, Korean, and Chinese increased dramatically (U.S. Bureau of the Census, 1990). The number of languages spoken in each U.S. state varies widely (Baker and Jones, 1998). R. Bravo (personal communication,

March, 2001), at the U.S. Bureau of the Census, expected the number of speakers of languages other than English to increase. Language demographics from the 2000 Census, first available in the summer of 2002, will post to the website http://factfinder.census.gov.

The percentages of people in the 1990 U.S. Census speaking languages other than English and who reported not speaking English well or at all are listed in Table 1.3 (see page 12) for the top 10 spoken languages in the United States. Approximately 20% of those who speak one of the top 10 languages currently spoken in the United States reported that they did not speak English fluently.

Information on English language proficiency of school-aged children has implications for assessment and intervention. There are a total of 2,308,038 English language learner (ELL) students in the United States. The numbers and percentages of ELLs (i.e., students whose primary language is not English) enrolled in kindergarten through grade 12 in the United States are reported in Table 1.4 (see page 13) for the top 10 languages (Fleischman and Hopstock, 1993).

The number of ELL students for the 1999–2000 school year was projected to be as high 4,148,997—a 104.3% increase in enrollment from 1989–1990 (National Clearinghouse for Bilingual Education, 1999). Five states provided the residency for approximately 67% of all ELL students: California (30%), Texas (15%), New York (11%), Florida (6%), and Illinois (5%) (August and Hakuta, 1998). With so many diverse languages and the movement of various linguistic groups in the United States

11

Table 1.3

Speakers of the Top 10 Languages Other than English Reporting Lack of Fluency in English

Rank	Language	Total (U.S. Census-1990)	Number of speakers reportedly not fluent in English	Percentage of speakers reportedly non-fluent in English	Rank in nonfluency
	TOTAL	31,844,979	6,672,201	20.9%	
1	Spanish	17,339,172	4,500,973	25.9	4
2	French	1,702,176	157,724	9.26	8
3	German	1,547,099	101,163	6.56	10
4	Italian	1,308,648	151, 262	11.55	7
5	Chinese	1,249, 213	373,296	29.88	2
6	Tagalog	843,251	63,028	7.47	9
7	Polish	743,251	98,384	13.23	6
8	Korean	626,478	188,419	30.07	1
9	Vietnamese	507,069	143,173	28.23	3
10	Portuguese	429,860	98,334	22.87	5

Source: U.S. Bureau of the Census (1990)

and around the globe, there is an increasing need for individuals who can help bridge the linguistic barrier between individuals who cannot communicate in the same language.

Table 1.4

**Ten Most Common Languages
Other than English Spoken by K–12
English Language Learners (ELLs)**

Rank	Language	Number of ELL students	Percent
1	Spanish	1,682,560	72.9%
2	Vietnamese	90,922	3.9
3	Hmong	42,305	1.8
4	Cantonese	38,693	1.7
5	Cambodian	37,742	1.6
6	Korean	36,568	1.6
7	Laotian	29,838	1.3
8	Navajo	28,913	1.3
9	Tagalog	24,516	1.1
10	Russian	21,903	0.9

Source: Fleischman and Hopstock (1993)

THE NEED FOR INTERPRETERS AND TRANSLATORS

Collaboration with an interpreter or translator is a necessity when the speech-language pathologist or audiologist does not share a common language with the client. The number of languages spoken in some communities across the United States exceeds 100 (Bracken and McCallum, 2001). Even though an increase in the number of certified bilingual speech-language pathologists and audiologists has been noted in the last 20 years or so, their languages may not match those of their clients or they may not be available in rural or other areas of the country. Approximately 2,000 members of the American Speech-Language-Hearing Association (ASHA)—or 2% of the entire membership of 100,000—reported that they provide services in languages other than English (S. Martínez, personal communication, September 7, 1999).

The Individuals with Disabilities Education Act (IDEA) (1997) and most state special education laws require that assessment be in a student's native language "unless it is clearly not feasible to do so" (§ 614 [a] [3] [A] [ii]). The laws do not specify that intervention must be provided in the student's native language. They do, however, specify that written notices and descriptions of procedural safeguards must be provided in the family's primary language "unless it is clearly not feasible to do so" (§ 615 [b] [4]). Therefore, collaborating with an interpreter or translator who is fluent in English and in the student's primary language is necessary to provide appropriate special education services. Some states have more stringent requirements. For example, Title 5 Section 3023 of the California Education Code states:

> Assessments shall be administered by qualified personnel who are competent in both the oral or sign language skills and written skills of the individual's primary language or mode of communication and have a knowledge and understanding of the cultural and ethnic background of the pupil. If it clearly is not feasible to do so, an interpreter must be used, and the assessment report shall document this condition and note that the validity of the assessment may have been affected.

Traditionally, people performing the duties of an interpreter or translator in speech, language, and hearing have been bilingual with a variety of educational backgrounds and levels of training. A report from 18 school districts in California indicated that the services of bilingual speech-language pathology assistants were used to help with assessments, to provide direct language services to monolingual preschool students who came from primarily Spanish-speaking backgrounds, and to communicate with parents. An unspecified number of districts provided in-service training for the support personnel who performed the duties of

> [B]ilingual assistants were trained by the speech-language pathologist with whom they worked.

an interpreter or translator. The report concluded that, for the most part, these bilingual assistants were trained by the speech-language pathologist with whom they worked (California Speech-Language-Hearing Association, 1997). More detailed research on how interpreters or translators collaborate with ASHA members is not currently available (S. Martínez, personal communication, July, 2000).

METHODS OF INTERPRETING AND TRANSLATING

There are two basic methods of interpreting: consecutive and simultaneous. In *consecutive interpreting*, the message is translated into the second language once it is spoken in the first lan-

15

guage. This results in a short lag time between when the message is spoken and when it is heard. Consecutive interpreting is the most common method used in educational or clinical settings. It provides more personal communication because the interaction takes place among a small group of people.

In *simultaneous interpreting*, the message is translated without any lag time since the message is conveyed in the first language at the same time as it is interpreted in the second. Simultaneous interpreting is most commonly used at international conferences. It may be used in an educational or clinical setting when a conference necessitates sharing a great deal of information or where there are many specialists present. In these instances, the interpreter may whisper the interpretation to the speakers of the second language to maintain the flow of the meeting as others are speaking.

There are two basic methods of translation: prepared and sight. In a *prepared translation* method, the written translation of a given document, such as a letter, a report, or an IEP, is prepared in advance. In a *sight translation*, a written document is translated orally at the same time the document is read. In communication disorders settings, the prepared method is more common.

Helpful Resources

Few resources describe the roles of bilingual support personnel working with speech-language pathologists or audiologists. Procedures have been based on practices developed in other fields employing interpreters and translators and have not been validated in speech-language pathology, audiology, and related fields like psychological assessment or counseling. The following materials may guide the development of education and research programs for interpreters and translators:

Cheng, L.L., Langdon, H.W., and Davies, D. (1991). *The art of interpreting: A dynamic process* [Video]. San Diego, CA: Department of Communication Disorders, San Diego State University.

Langdon, H.W. (2000). *Assessment of English learners with the collaboration of an interpreter/translator* [Video]. San José, CA: San José State University.

Langdon, H.W. (2002). *Interpreters and translators in communication disorders: A practitioner's handbook.* Eau Claire, WI: Thinking Publications.

Langdon, H.W., Siegel, V., Halog, L., and Sánchez-Boyce, M. (1994). *Interpreter translator manual in the educational setting.* Sacramento, CA: Resources in Special Education.

2 Communicating in a Multilingual Society

Code-switching is sometimes wrongly perceived as a haphazard process and a sign of linguistic incompetence.

—*Colin Baker and Sylvia Prys Jones*

Chapter Goals

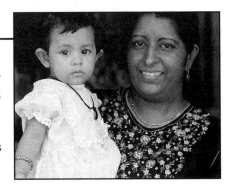

- Explain how phonology, grammar, semantics, and pragmatics affect dialect

- Describe normal patterns of code switching

- Delineate the causes of language loss

- Identify how code switching and language loss relate to the interpreting and translating process

- Discuss the clinical applications of code switching and language loss

DISCUSSION ITEMS

1. What information might an interpreter provide about the grammar of a client's primary language?

2. How could inattention to nonverbal communication interfere with the success of a family conference?

3. What are some of the semantic variations within a language that an interpreter should be aware of?

4. How would you explain to a colleague that code switching is not an indication of weak linguistic skills?

5. How can an interpreter help a speech-language pathologist or audiologist determine if a client is experiencing language loss?

6. When would code switching by the interpreter not be appropriate?

7. What information should be collected in a classroom observation to assist in determining if a student's code switching is within expectations?

DIALECTS

Multiple dialects may be spoken in a given region or country. The distinction between a language and a dialect is not always clear. Regional dialects of English or Spanish are easily identified as being one united language because, other than differences in pronunciation and some vocabulary, these dialects are mutually intelligible. Individuals who speak Puerto Rican Spanish, for example, find themselves using very different words from speakers of Mexican or Castilian Spanish, but they can still communicate. In other cases, even when dialects are mutually intelligible, they are regarded as separate languages for political reasons. For example, Swedish, Danish, Norwegian, and Icelandic are mutually intelligible and could be considered dialects of the same language, but, for political reasons, they are each considered different languages. The opposite can occur as well. Different varieties or dialects of Chinese are mutually unintelligible, but they are considered to be the same language (Crystal, 1997). Languages and regional dialects vary in phonology, grammar, semantics, and pragmatics. Some broad characteristics of each parameter are described in the following sections.

Phonology

Phonology includes the study of speech sounds in a language. Phonological differences (i.e., pronunciation) across languages and dialects account for languages' most noticeable characteristics. Phonological differences in dialects may manifest themselves through phonemes that are pronounced differently across languages. Conversely, the elimination of contrasts

21

between basic phonemes is also common. For example, American English "pin" and "pen" are pronounced the same in the regional dialects of the Midwest United States (Cheng, 1994a). Phonological variations may also occur as a result of contact with other dialects or languages.

Nilsen and Nilsen (1973) provided a useful list of the English vowel and consonant contrasts that may cause difficulty to speakers of various languages. For example, speakers of Arabic, Finnish, Italian, and Tagalog may have difficulty differentiating contrasts between /I/ and /e/ as in "hid" and "head" or "chick" and "check." The contrasts between /v/ and /θ/ as in "vat" and "that" may be difficult for speakers of Arabic, Burmese, Dutch, Hindi, Navajo, Polish, Russian, Tagalog, and Vietnamese.

Audiologists should be aware that performance on tasks requiring discrimination of minimal pairs (i.e., words that vary by only one phoneme) may be affected by a client's language or dialect. Likewise, speech-language pathologists may compare transcriptions of an interpreter's pronunciation of items with a client's pronunciation in determining a possible speech disorder. However, speech-language pathologists must also consider the possibility of dialectical variations in each person's production of speech sounds.

Grammar

Grammar is the system of rules for combining words and word parts into sentences. Throughout history, languages have undergone continual change reflecting two levels of grammatical variation: (1) the formation of words from meaningful units of the language (morphology) and (2) the combination of words into larger structures, such as phrases and sentences (syntax). Variations exist in word class, sentence structure, arrangement of structure, and word placement within phrases. Verbs, verb auxiliaries, negatives, inflectional suffixes in nouns, various forms of pronouns, articles, and adverbs all undergo variation over time.

Language structures can vary significantly between languages. The use of loan words is common and acceptable in some languages (e.g., *retirarse* [to retire] is used rather than the Spanish verb *jubilarse)*. In contrast, certain

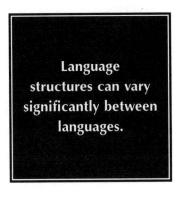

Language structures can vary significantly between languages.

languages such as Japanese, Tibetan, Korean, and Javanese use honorific forms (i.e., forms that show respect) and loan words or dialectal variations are expressly avoided when addressing certain people. The grammatical forms used for different degrees of politeness change, as do first- and second-person pronouns. Several European languages make the distinction between two forms of *you* (e.g., the Spanish *tú* and *usted,* the French *tu* and *vous,* the German *du* and *zie,* and the Polish *ty* and *pan* for masculine or *pani* for feminine). For further examples of specific forms, see Crystal (1997).

Interpreters can provide important information about the grammatical systems of speakers. Grammatical rules in a speaker's native language may be misapplied to English and could be misinterpreted by the communication disorders professional as part of a language-development difficulty. For example, a grammatical feature that does not exist in the speaker's first language may be used when not expected in English. Interpreters can identify patterns of grammatical errors that may be observed in the speaker's native language productions.

Semantics

Semantics is the study of word meanings. All words have recognized meanings. These meanings are not static, but change over time. Some words change their meanings completely and take on different cultural twists. Furthermore, the sociocultural events that are associated with the words may not be readily translucent to all communicators. For example, in the United States, when someone asks if he or she can buy somebody a drink, it usually means an alcoholic beverage, not milk or soda. In other cultures, nonalcoholic beverages would be included in the reference.

Originally, the study of semantics focused on vocabulary. However, because words undergo continual changes due to language use, it is difficult to separate words from their context. Words can have a different meaning as a result of prosody, for example. The meaning changes in the sentences "I want to buy the yellow *roses"* (difference between roses and other flowers) and "I want to buy the *yellow* roses" (difference between yellow and another color). The setting in which a sentence is spoken is another way that context changes the meaning of a word. For example, "the door is open" may signal that a person can come in or that the door needs to be closed. Some word changes may be introduced or used by specific segments of the population, like teens or young adults. Other changes occur as a result of scientific progress, like technology or medicine, or from contact with other languages within a given community. For example, the influence of English on Spanish has created many Anglicized words such as *lonchear* (to have lunch) rather than *almorzar, parquear* (to park) rather than *estacionarse*, and *retirarse* (to retire) rather than *jubilarse*.

Semantic variations are important considerations for interpreters and translators. When words or phrases are directly translated to their dictionary meanings, the intended meaning of the speaker may be lost. Interpreters must be aware of intonation and other cues for meaning. Speakers with different language dialects also vary their use of vocabulary. Interpreters should seek clarification when a word seems to be used incongruously.

Pragmatics

Pragmatics refers to the relationship between signs or linguistic expressions and their use in a sociolinguistic context. Content, social setting, connotation, inflection, and intonation play a role in the transmission of meaning in communication. Note that many of these items are nonverbal. Distinctions between literal and nonliteral meaning, nuance, and innuendo may be lost or misinterpreted in a cross-cultural setting where two communicators perceive a situation differently. One of the essential roles of language is to establish and maintain social interaction (Crystal, 1997). The social context and the relationship between participants are crucial to conversation. Several steps are

> Content, social setting, connotation, inflection, and intonation play a role in the transmission of meaning in communication.

25

Pragmatics and Bilingualism

Kallen (2000) suggested that excessive attention to the structural aspects of language (i.e., phonology, grammar, and semantics) interferes with the ability to understand the concept of bilingualism. To appreciate the pragmatics involved in bilingualism, it is necessary to pay attention to nine items:

1. Textual/Pragmatic—what speakers do with different codes and registers in sustained discourse and a variety of media

2. Cultural—the values that are attached to and expressed by language

3. Social—the social and professional status each speaker holds and how these are reflected in the use of one or the other language

4. Evaluative—the attitudes toward self, others, context, and language the speakers hold in using one or another language in different situations

5. Cognitive—the relationship that exists between language and thinking

6. Use—what can be done by using a given language

7. Variation across languages—the significance that exists in the speaker's use of code switching (i.e., use of two languages in a conversation), diglossia (i.e., use of two languages), or intralanguage variations (e.g., register, style, and dialect)

> **Pragmatics and Bilingualism—***Continued*
>
> 8. Identity—the degree to which the language represents or shapes the speaker's concept of self
>
> 9. Valorization—the value attached to a given language as part of a social context

involved in the communication process: selection of a topic, initiation of speech, turn taking, maintenance of the topic, and closure of the conversation (Wolfram and Christian, 1989).

Nonverbal communication is also a component of pragmatics. Chapter 3 reviews the importance of nonverbal communication and its components, which are vital to a successful exchange between two parties whether or not they share the same language (see "Nonverbal Aspects," page 46). The nonverbal aspect of this exchange becomes even more important when two parties do not share the same language and collaboration with an interpreter is necessary.

CODE SWITCHING AND LANGUAGE LOSS

Code Switching

The majority of the world's population is bilingual (Baker and Jones, 1998). As Crystal (1997) stated, "multilingualism is the natural way of life for hundreds of millions all over the world....it is obvious that an enormous amount of language contact must be taking place" (p. 362). When bilingual individuals interact, they code switch (i.e., change languages within a conversation). This is a common and normal phenomenon (Hong, Morris, Chiu, and Benet-Martínez, 2000; Myers-Scotton, 1992). Speech-language pathologists, audiologists, and related professionals who work with bilingual populations must be cognizant of code switching.

Code switching is the general term used whenever a conversation includes two languages with a switch from one language to the other occurring at the word, phrase, or sentence level (Poplack, 1980). However, code switching has been given several definitions, depending on the particular part of speech or discourse considered. Gumpertz (1982) defined it as "the juxtaposition within the same speech exchange of passages of speech belonging to different grammatical systems or subsystems" (p. 59). According to Poplack (1980), code switching is the alternate use of two languages.

Code mixing is a more specific term that indicates that a word in the alternate language has been used within a given sentence (e.g., "dame el spoon" for "give me the spoon"). Code mixing occurs when the beginning of the sentence is started in one language (e.g., English) and the end of the sentence is verbalized in the other (e.g., French) for example, "Come here, je veux te montrer quelque chose" for "Come here, I want to show you something".

Until the last 20 years, code switching was believed to result from an individual's inability to converse effectively in either of two languages. Terms such as *Spanglish, Tex-Mex, Franglais,* or

Hinglish have been used to denote the alternate use of two languages within a conversation. These terms have often been used in a derogatory manner. In some bilingual communities, code switching has been purposefully avoided so that the communities may not be negatively targeted (Baker and Jones, 1998). In the past, terms such as *code mixing, interference,* and *borrowing,* were used to imply a negative value judgement about the sophistication of the speaker's language use. It is now clear, however, that code switching is a communication strategy used by proficient bilingual speakers.

> **Code switching is a common phenomenon, and the most competent bilingual speakers switch from one language to another.**

All over the world bilinguals carry on such conversations...in every nation, successful business people and professionals who happen to have a different home language from the dominant language in the society where they live, frequently engage in code-switching (between these two languages) with friends and business associates who share their linguistic repertoires. (Myers-Scotton, 1993, p. 17)

Code switching is a common phenomenon, and the most competent bilingual speakers switch from one language to another during a given conversation. Bilingual individuals learn to use code switching as a strategy to facilitate more effective communication with family members, peers, and other conversational partners (Cheng and Butler, 1989). Bilingual speakers are often unaware that they are switching languages as they converse. Alternating from one language to the other can occur between utterances within a single conversational turn or within the same utterance (Milroy and Muysken, 1995). Code switching may serve various purposes, including:

- Emphasizing a given point

- Relating something that was learned or occurred while using the alternate language

- Accessing words in the alternate language when there are no equivalent words in the language of interaction (e.g., words like *quinceañera* or *bat mitzvah,* which have specific cultural connotations)

- Expressing a specific feeling or emotion that is connected to the alternate language

- Interjecting humor into a conversation

- Excluding someone from participating in a conversation

(Myers-Scotton, 1992)

Research Findings

Research is concentrating on identifying specific situations in which code switching occurs. For example, Martin-Jones (1995) conducted several classroom observations where bilingual assistants were participating in the instructional process. She noted that each language was used for different purposes. English was used when the assistant was emphasizing some key concepts, but the native language was used when directions were given. Thus, there was a difference between "curriculum talk" and "learner talk." More research of this nature is needed to understand when languages are switched and for what purposes.

Code switching is also a common phenomenon occurring in early bilingualism. Bilingual children who are in the process of acquiring two languages can switch back and forth according to the context. They are very aware of when to change the language they speak according to the situation. For example, they know to speak one language with one parent and the other language with the other parent. There are reports that children might use the opposite language in a given moment to attract attention from either parent (Bergman, 1976; Goodz, 1994; Leopold, 1970; Ronjat, 1913). Langdon and Merino (1992) conducted a thorough review of this topic.

Such use of two languages may be called code switching only if it does not violate a syntactic rule.

Another type of code switching may occur when a child infuses the two languages within the same sentence or a given word. An example is that of a child's use of the prefix of one language and the ending of another within the same word, as in the following situation. When a bilingual Spanish- and Polish-speaking child said to his sister, "Jéchame más," using the root of Polish *jechacz* meaning *to drive* and the suffix *me* for the Spanish imperative (making the phrase "Drive me"), the sister responded, "Ya te jeché bastante" ("I have driven you enough"), again using the Polish verb *jechacz* within a Spanish sentence (Langdon and Merino, 1992).

Such use of two languages may be called code switching

only if it does not violate a syntactic rule of a given language. For example, when conversing in English and French, it would be permissible to say, "Elle est allée au mall," with the switch between the subject and object, but not, "She est allée au mall," with the switch between the subject pronoun and the verb (Baker and Jones, 1998, p. 61). For speech-language pathologists and audiologists interested in specific rules of code switching, Milroy and Muysken (1995) offer a series of articles on various subjects related to code switching in their collection.

Language Loss

When two or more languages are used by a speaker, proficiency in the lesser used language may decline over time. Several social, personal, cultural, and linguistic reasons contribute to this phenomenon. Political and social reasons include reduced number of speakers in a given geographical area, distance from the country where the language is spoken, greater use of the majority language that is required for employment, general lack of opportunity to use the native language, and an individual's belief that social and vocational promotion will not occur unless the native language is dropped.

Personal reasons may result when a spouse or a partner does not share the language. If only one spouse speaks a given language, he or she may not have opportunities to speak it with people outside the immediate family. Therefore, the couple's children are less likely to learn and use the language. For example, one of the authors grew up speaking Polish in Mexico and used the language to communicate with parents, grandparents, and friends of the family, but not peers. Currently, she uses only

Polish to communicate with her parents and a few friends. Thus, the author's child no longer comprehends or uses the language. The use of Polish within the family will eventually be lost.

Cultural factors that cause language loss include greater use of the majority language for cultural and religious events. Increased education and more acceptance of the majority language may also lead to language loss.

There are many linguistic factors that contribute to language loss. These include unavailability of the native language in a written form, an individual's beliefs that the native language has no international importance, and illiteracy in the native language (Baker and Jones, 1998; Edwards, 1994).

> Speech-language pathologists must consider language loss in assessing a client's proficiency in the native language.

Speech-language pathologists must consider language loss in assessing a client's proficiency in the native language. Verifying the frequency and quality of language used in the native language assists in determining if lack of proficiency is caused by less opportunity to interact with the language or be exposed to the language. For example, a client may not perform as well in certain areas like reading or writing in the native language because formal instruction in the language has not been consistent or has not been available. The client may not know certain concepts in the native language due to lack of exposure or practice. Therefore, taking a detailed history of language use is important in determining whether language loss might be the result of a language impairment instead of a language loss (Langdon and Merino, 1992).

Applications to the Interpreting and Translating Process

There are times in the interpreting process that interpreters may code switch when the participants have at least receptive knowledge of the two languages. They may code switch when there is not an equivalent word or concept in the other language. Depending on the situation, the impact of not knowing the exact word may or may not be important. Much depends on the context in which the interpreting or translating is occurring.

Interference between two languages may also occur because of similarities between words in the two languages (Gile, 1995). For example, there might be a temptation to interpret "she is embarrassed" as "está embarazada" (which actually means "she is pregnant"). Interference is common when words are similar across languages, especially during sight translation when words are translated in the same order across languages. For example, when translating a title from English, such *as Special Education Rights of Parents and Children,* it is tempting to do a word-by-word translation instead of shifting the word order of the phrase to *Derechos de los padres y los niños en relación con la educación especial* (Rights of Parents and Children in Relation to Education Special).

Interpreters need to be aware of their own potential language loss if they have inadequate opportunities to use a particular language. Moreover, since living languages continually change, interpreters need to remain current with new vocabulary and other linguistic changes.

Clinical Applications

Speech-language pathologists, audiologists, interpreters, and translators need to be aware of code switching as they work together in the assessment and intervention process with bilingual children and adults. Clearly, more data are needed to understand the linguistic and social constraints of code switching during oral communication (code switching during written translation is rare and usually inappropriate, unless a particular word is not translatable [e.g., bat mitzvah].) Possible language loss must also be considered during assessment. With advances in understanding these common linguistic phenomena, clinicians need to make a more detailed analysis of the nature of code switching and language loss. For professionals who work with children, observing classroom or social interactions and conversing with family members are important activities to help determine if a student's language patterns reflect those they hear and use at home or in the classroom. Many professionals will also work with brain-injured individuals. To date, studies on code switching patterns in bilingual adults who sustained brain injuries is almost nonexistent. Reyes (1995) reported that the few existing studies indicate that those adults' code switching patterns correspond to the patterns noted premorbidly.

Narrative assessment can be a tool for evaluating language use, including code switching and language loss. A *narrative* is an organizer of human experiences consisting of a form with a unique sequence of events containing the essence of the message and the speaker's communicative intent (Silliman and Diehl, 1995). The use of narratives demands a degree of cognitive and linguistic ability for its construction. A narrative is an account of happenings from a wide range of human experiences common in all languages, and there is a general consensus that narrative assessment is an important part of language assessment. However, the construction of narrative varies across cultures and languages, and this must be taken into account (Berman and Slobin, 1994; Hughes, McGillivray, and Schmidek, 1997; Westby and Roman, 1995).

Comparing the patterns used by a student with those used by others in the student's classroom and home would assist in determining if there might be a language impairment. Using mediated instruction and focusing on communication in one language at a time would assist the clinician in determining an effective instructional approach. Those students who need more coaching and repetition may be exhibiting a language-learning difficulty. Both the speech-language pathologist or audiologist and the interpreter need to be aware of code switching in the narratives of bilingual individuals.

Research efforts have also been directed to narrative studies in bilingual children with language impairments (Gutiérrez-Clellen, Peña, and Quinn, 1995). The information and observations provided in this study suggest that one method of determining whether or not the amount of code switching is greater than would be expected is to observe how the two languages are utilized in the instructional process.

The Code-Switching Forum, available through the Internet (http://groups.yahoo.com/group/code-switching), enables interested people to keep up with the emergence of new information and research data. The forum is an unmoderated list for discussion of code switching, bilingual conversation, and related phenomena.

3 Balancing Linguistic and Cultural Variables

To speak another language is to lead a parallel life: the better you speak any language, the more fully you live in another culture.

—*Barbara Wilson*

Chapter Goals

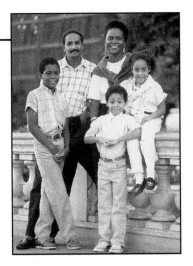

- Discuss the many areas that hold challenges for interpreters and translators, including verbal, nonverbal, cultural, and contextual areas

- Offer suggestions on how to respond to common questions that occur in the daily collaboration between a speech-language pathologist or audiologist and an interpreter or a translator

DISCUSSION ITEMS

1. What can the communication disorders professional do in his or her verbal communication to facilitate effective interpreting?

2. What methods could a communication disorders professional and interpreter use to make sure they are not overlooking or misunderstanding nonverbal communication from a client?

3. Use the continuum of cultural competence on page 50 to determine the level of competence currently expressed in your workplace or other familiar setting. What observations have you made that support this determination?

4. How would you explain these situations to a client or family member who is unfamiliar with medical, educational, and legal systems in the United States?

   - The roles of an audiologist versus an otolaryngologist

   - A medical procedure and the need for signed consent

   - Parent and child rights in special education

   - Placement in a special education program

5. Select a question and answer from pages 55–60. Role-play a situation in which the question and answer occurs.

CHALLENGES FOR INTERPRETERS

Speech-language pathologists and audiologists must remember that the responsibilities of interpreters extend far beyond conveying words from one language to another. The process entails bringing together two different voices so that linguistic and cultural differences will no longer constitute a barrier to communication. This idea is expressed in the following statement:

> When I pull a few cassettes from the carton beneath my desk and listen to random snatches, I am plunged into a pungent wash of remembrance and, at the same time, I am reminded of the lessons I am still learning from both of the cultures I have written about. Now and then when I play the tapes at night, I imagine what they would sound like if I could somehow splice them together, so the voices of the Hmong and voices of the American doctors could be heard on a single tape, speaking a common language. (Fadiman, 1997, p. ix)

[T]he responsibilities of interpreters extend far beyond conveying words from one language to another.

The interpreting process is far from simple—despite careful interpretation and consideration of cultural variables, something might be lost. Tan (1989) brought up this notion very clearly:

> I began to write stories using all the Englishes I grew up with: the English I spoke to my mother, which for

lack of a better term might be described as 'simple', the English she used with me, which for lack of a better term might be described as 'broken'; my translation of her Chinese, which could certainly be described as 'watered down', and what I imagined to be her translation of her Chinese if she could speak in perfect English, her internal language and for which I sought to preserve the essence, neither an English nor a Chinese structure. (p. 32)

Some schools of thought advocate that the role of interpreters should be limited to conveying meaning rather than assisting in bridging two cultures (Penney and Sammons, 1997). But, in reality, the interpreter is the only person in the typical triad of the client, service provider, and interpreter who understands the messages as they are conveyed the first time around by each party. The interpreter is also at the center of the turn-taking process (Englund Dimitrova, 1997). In addition, the interpreter is the one who ultimately negotiates the speaking time, indicating to each party that the message might be too long, complex, or unclear to convey in the other language. The dynamics of the process require that the interpreter attend to both verbal and nonverbal communication signals. To be successful, the interpreter must understand the context of the interaction. For example, a different discourse takes place when a speech-language pathologist asks specific questions about a child's language development as compared to when a parent is given program options for a child or when an audiologist describes the properties and uses of a given hearing aid. In essence, the role of the interpreter is not only to focus on the linguistic aspect of the interaction but also on the communication itself. As Gentile (1997) indicated, it is necessary to differentiate "interpreter" from "interpreting." The interpreter is not like a machine that conveys word-by-word renditions; the emotion and tone of the original message must be maintained, even if offensive or vulgar (Nicholson and Martinsen, 1997).

Breakdowns in communication occur when the conversational participants make erroneous interpretations about each other's meaning and intent. Language is embedded in people's history and culture. Therefore, understanding the history, culture, and socialization patterns of a given group is crucial in securing cross-cultural communicative competence. True communicative competence in a second language requires an ability to integrate language, culture, history, social knowledge, and cognition. As Hall (1977) so aptly said, "All [cultures] have their own identity, language systems of nonverbal communication, material culture, history and *ways of doing things*" (p. 2).

> The interpreter
> is not like a machine
> that conveys
> word-by-word
> renditions.

Challenges in interpretation and translation include idiomatic expressions, emotional connotation of words, and humor. Probably one of the last aspects of culture to be understood by a second language learner is the emotional and even legalistic implications of a given word in a certain situation. This aspect was exemplified in the dispute between the United States and China regarding the loss of a military plane in early 2001. The word *sorry* was translated into Chinese as *yihan*, which did not carry the connotation of guilt. Instead *sorry* or *regret* should have been translated as *bao qian,* which renders the more apologetic tone that was expected by the Chinese (Smith, 2001).

Effective communication between two parties mediated by an interpreter is often difficult to achieve for several reasons, particularly those related to training issues. In some cases, interpreters have not received any formal training and in others the training has been inconsistent. The philosophy of what constitutes effective interpreting in specific settings (e.g., medical or educational) has not been defined. The lack of recognition for interpreters working in educational settings is frequently mentioned (Carr, 1997). Another reason is the lack of consensus regarding the role of interpreting (i.e., the dilemma about the role of the interpreter as conveyer of meaning or mediator of communication). The interpreter must simultaneously balance four different variables—verbal, nonverbal, cultural, and contextual—to achieve successful communication in two different languages. The interaction among these components is represented in Figure 3.1.

Verbal Aspects

The verbal component of the interpretation process requires understanding, visualizing, and recreating the message in the target language (Gile, 1995). Furthermore, specialized training may be required to translate to and from particular languages. Researchers who have focused on this issue have different opinions. Some feel that the process is universal, others that it

The Interpreter's Role in the
Figure 3.1 **Communication Process**

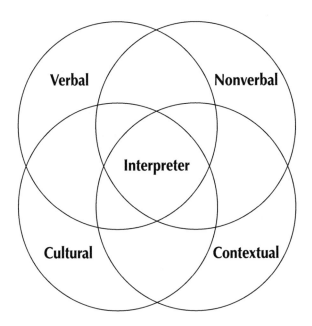

is language specific. For example, interpreting from French to German might require different skills than interpreting from Japanese to English. Gile (1986) reported that certain words in Japanese are pronounced identically, but may have different meanings, so the challenge in interpreting Japanese is greater than it is for many other languages. He further noted that for a long time, researchers have neglected looking at the specificity of language and have masked the process with other than purely linguistic issues, such as attention and memory. It is time to analyze the linguistic aspect more carefully.

In a typical discourse, "the number of grammatical structures that emerge (given a specific context, in this case, the process of assessment and assessment itself) is finite and...what really varies is the lexicon" (Gile, 1995, p.213). Content words, such as nouns, verbs, adjectives, and adverbs, are carriers of information and differ across languages in length and phonetic richness. Vocabulary shows essential differences because it reflects what is important in that language (Lustig and Koester, 1999). Specific linguistic features remind us about differences within members of a given group. For example, as stated earlier, in Spanish there are two types of *you*, and in many Asian languages, several different forms of *you* are used depending on who is addressed. Some languages may have very specific words to denote specific variations or subtleties for a concept. However, a talented interpreter can find a way to render the concept in an alternate language when there is no equivalent word for it.

The process of interpreting is challenging because some structures are definitely more difficult to translate. For example, embedded sentences (e.g., "The boy whose ball was caught in the net had a yellow shirt that was torn") can put a heavy demand on short-term memory skills.

In other instances, decisions about which words to use might be challenging due to possible cross-linguistic interference. For example, "library" is interpreted into French as "bibliothèque," while the French "libraire" means "bookstore." *Cartoons* and *cartones*, two nouns that share similar configurations, are different words: "cartoons" should be interpreted as the Spanish "caricaturas." Similarly, idioms cannot be interpreted into other languages easily because of their linguistic or cultural specificity (Baker and Jones, 1998). Examples include:

"It's Greek to me!"

French: "It is Chinese to me!" (C'est du chinois)

"Give him an inch and he'll take a mile!"

Spanish: "You give him (or her) a hand and he (or she) grabs the foot!" (Le da la mano y se toma el pie)

"Go jump in the lake!"

Hebrew: "Go whistle in the ocean!" (Gai feifen ahfe-nayam)

When one of the parties has an accent in a given language that might interfere with smooth communication, or when a child or an adult has a speech-language impairment, the process of interpreting becomes even more challenging. A speaker's accent may unjustly convey a negative

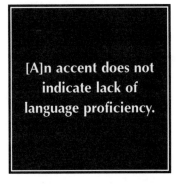

[A]n accent does not indicate lack of language proficiency.

impression on native speakers of a given language. Unfortunately, the perception of accents varies from listener to listener: some people may react neutrally, others negatively. All speakers, however, have an accent. Speech-language pathologists, audiologists, interpreters, and translators should remember that an accent does not indicate lack of language proficiency. Langdon (1999) discussed in greater detail the influence of accent and its implication for clinical practice. The role of the interpreter is further complicated because there might be differences in the parties' educational levels, and, therefore, in their usage of words. Also, a client's perception of an interpreter may depend on the interpreter's accent, which may influence the client's trust in the process. Thus, the interpreter needs to "manipulate a large spectrum of speech styles from the most formal and articulate to the least coherent nonstandard variety in two languages" (Benmaman, 1997, p. 184).

Interpretation is also complex because many words include two types of meanings. The *denotative meaning* carries the public, objective, and legal meaning of a given word. The *connotative meaning* carries more of the personal, emotionally charged, private meaning (Lustig and Koester, 1999).

Nonverbal Aspects

There is no question that every communication act contains a nonverbal component. Knapp (1972) indicated that less than 35% of a message's social meaning is transmitted through words alone, whereas 65% of that social meaning is conveyed through nonverbal communication. Scollon and Scollon (1995) described three specific aspects of nonverbal communication that are relevant to intercultural communication: the movements of our bodies (kinesis), our use of space (proxemics), and our use of time (monochronic or polychronic). Two individuals using different linguistic codes (e.g., English and Spanish) differ in how they apply the sociocultural rules related to these three aspects. Unfortunately, as Gile (1995) stated:

> There are no formal sets of rules to provide a systematic list of the meanings of a culture's nonverbal code systems. But, we cannot ignore that nonverbal messages

can be used to accent, complement, contradict, regulate, or substitute for the verbal message. (p. 226)

Although the display of emotions and other nonverbal communication traits may seem to be universal, their use and their interpretation may vary from culture to culture. There is universality in the facial expressions of happiness, sadness, fear, surprise, anger, and disgust (Burgoon, Buller, and Woodall, 1996). Specifically, Ekman (1975) found that fear is indicated by a furrowed brow, raised eyebrows, wide-open eyes, creased or pinched base of the nose, taut cheeks, partially open mouth, and upturned upper lip. On the other hand, a smile is often interpreted differently cross-culturally, including embarrassment, friendliness, or warning of tension (Lustig and Koester, 1999). Lack of eye contact in Latino and Asian cultures shows respect but may be interpreted to mean the opposite in European cultures. Likewise, more touching prevails in Latino cultures compared to Germanic or Japanese cultures (Lustig and Koester, 1999). Thus, despite similarities in the ways in which humans use and understand different signals, many of those signals are modified by cultural interpretation. In addition, vocal expression displays different emotions through variations in loudness and pitch, but some of these variations are culture bound. For example, Arabs and North Americans often use louder voices compared to Britons and continental Europeans (Burgoon et al. 1996).

Many nonverbal messages, like facial expressions and tone of voice, are not explicitly taught but are learned through observation or personal experience within a given culture. In addition, there might be age, gender, and personality differences that vary from individual to individual. When one speaks a given language, one can more readily associate the verbal and non-verbal components (Brislin, 1981). However, this synchrony is unfamiliar to the party who does not know a given language. Part of the interpreter's role is to manage two languages that depend on two different verbal and nonverbal messages.

Speech-language pathologists and audiologists should remind interpreters to transmit nonverbal aspects of an individual's communication. This information may have important implications for assessment and intervention.

Cultural Aspects

The acquisition of cultural competence involves not only the understanding of two cultures but also the acquisition of social and pragmatic knowledge. In other words, it is knowing what to say to whom, where, and when. Hall (1976), in his book *Beyond Culture,* clearly advocated for the need to cultivate such competence. As people face a shrinking world and globalization, they are compelled to communicate with people from linguistic and cultural backgrounds that are foreign. A culture is more than a group of people who share similar values, history, and language. It also refers to a group of people who share similar life experiences, a common world view, and similar patterns of social interaction. Without skills in cross-cultural negotiation, communication breakdown is inevitable. Those who mediate between cultures understand this concept very well.

Cultures differ greatly in their pragmatic rules. Thus, interpreters face challenges that go beyond form, function, and use of language (Cheng, 1998b, 1999). The interpreting process takes place in a structured situation where one of the speakers is the communication disorders professional and the other is the recipient (often from a culturally perceived less prestigious language). The interpreter is the participant who supposedly has command of both languages (Roy, 2000). Often, there is no social equality between the three participants, and neither the interpreter nor communication disorders professional may be properly trained to work with the other. As Englund Dimitrova (1997) indicated, very few people are used to or trained for communicating through another individual. In this situation, the interpreter becomes "the actor solving not only problems of translation, but problems of mutual understanding" (Roy, 2000, p. 30). Although the interpreter needs to remain neutral, the conversational flow must be maintained, and it is the interpreter who manages this flow. The success of the interpretation process is highly dependent on how the interpreter is able to coordinate the combination of verbal and nonverbal communication in two languages, a very complex task.

Essentially, the interpreter needs to convey the cultural knowledge and ways of speaking in a given situation and, "in the end all three participants jointly produce the event, and all three are responsible, in differing degrees for its communicative success or failure" (Roy, 2000, p. 100). The speech-language pathologist or audiologist should be mindful of the many demands on the interpreter and help in any way possible.

Communication disorders professionals should also be aware of the cultural beliefs that affect a family's reaction to a diagnosis or treatment recommendation. A cultural definition of what constitutes an impairment is critically dependent on the

Continuum of Cultural Competence

Cultural competence can be defined along a continuum of six levels, from destructive to full proficiency:

1. *Cultural destructiveness* is represented by attitudes, policies, and practices that are destructive to cultures and the individuals within the cultures.

2. *Cultural incapacity* is the lack of capacity to accept people who are different. The dominant culture remains extremely biased (e.g., discriminatory hiring practices and lower expectations).

3. *Cultural blindness* is a stage wherein color and culture make no difference and all people are considered to be the same. Cultural blindness ignores cultural strengths and encourages assimilation. There may be an unconscious assumption that people from different backgrounds are culturally deprived.

4. *Cultural precompetency* explores how to better work with diverse populations and attempts to improve some aspects of professional services.

5. *Cultural competency* accepts and respects differences, expands cultural knowledge, and provides a variety of adaptations of service models.

6. *Cultural proficiency* holds culture in high esteem and continues to add to the knowledge base.

(California State Department of Education, 1991)

values of each particular cultural group. However, differences exist even within a group, and the expected or anticipated reactions to disabilities can vary considerably. Some people may be relieved to obtain a diagnosis for a given speech, language, or hearing impairment, others may interpret the diagnosis negatively. For example, it is not unusual for certain Hispanic cultures to consider that an individual with such a diagnosis is also sick or retarded (Langdon, 1992a; Harry, 1992).

The treatment of birth defects and other disabilities is influenced by cultural beliefs and by the socioeconomic status of the individual and the family within a given group (Cheng, 1999; Gollnick and Chinn, 1990; Strauss, 1990). There are broad similarities and differences among Western and non-Western belief systems and practices. In all cultures, attitudes toward disabilities can be traced, in part, to folk beliefs and superstitions. A tendency exists to define the cause of a health-related problem in spiritual terms (Cheng, 1999; Meyerson, 1990; Strauss, 1990).

Many Eastern cultures view a disabling condition as the result of wrongdoing of the individual's ancestors, resulting in guilt and shame for the family. The cause of disabilities can be explained through a variety of spiritual and cultural beliefs, such as imbalance of inner forces, bad wind, spoiled foods, gods, demons or spirits, hot or cold forces, or fright. For example, the Chamorro culture (primarily on the island of Guam) views a disability as a gift from God and believes the disabled individual belongs to everyone. The disabled person is thus protected and sheltered by the family. Many Asian and Pacific Islanders believe that disability is caused by Karma (fate), and one can do nothing about it. Other cultures view disability as a curse, and many ostracize the individual from society (Cheng, 1989).

People from developed and developing regions of the world have different levels of education, exposure to cultures, and personal experiences. Attitudes toward disabilities are a reflection of current and historical beliefs about the nature of disabilities. All over the world, people use different methods to treat illnesses and diseases, including consulting with a priest, clansman, or elders before seeking the help of a licensed physician. Among the Hmong, for example, surgical intervention is viewed as harmful. Hmong believe that spirits may leave the body once the body is cut open, causing death (Fadiman, 1997). All over the world, treatments by healers range from medication or therapy, to acupuncture, massage, cao (coin rubbing), gat gio (pinching), giac (placing a very hot cup on the exposed area), steam inhalation, balm application, herbs, inhaling smoke or ashes from burnt incense, or the ingestion of hot or cold foods (Cheng, 1995). Other methods of healing include exercises such as Qi-Gong, over-the-counter drugs, prescription drugs, or a combination of methods. The variety of approaches and beliefs complicate the task of a western doctor who is unfamiliar with many of the practices and medications that may be used by a family. Such practices may be counter-productive when combined with the doctor's treatment.

> Attitudes toward disabilities are a reflection of current and historical beliefs.

Child-rearing practices and expectations of children also vary widely from culture to culture (Hammer and Weiss, 2000; Heath, 1983; van Kleeck, 1994; Westby, 1990). There are differences in how parents respond to their children's language, who interacts with children and how they interact, and how families encourage children to initiate and continue a verbal interaction. Socioeconomic and individual differences must always be considered as well as differences in educational practices. Some families understand and support bilingual education, others have no options or opinions because they believe that schools know best about how to educate their children. Among those families, there are a variety of attitudes toward the first and second language and culture, various levels of formal education in the first or second language, and differing expectations for their children (Butler and Cheng, 1996; Cheng, 1998; Hiebert, 1991). Communication disorders professionals have also found that cross-cultural differences affect family's perceptions of and reactions to assistive technology (Huer, 1997; Parette, Brotherson, and Huer, 2000).

Contextual Aspects

Different situations, or contexts, might determine the type of interpreting necessary, which in turn may or may not demand more skill on the part of the interpreter. Carr (1997) indicated that different levels of interpreting are necessary in the allied-health professions. For example, a straightforward interpretation is needed for an admission or interaction in a waiting room or hospital ward, while more complex knowledge is necessary for counseling, medical informed consents, and emergency situations. In a clinical setting, a complex situation would be where the interpreter needs to assist the speech-language pathologist in evaluating an individual who has a speech, language, or communication problem. Audiological counseling would also be difficult because of the need to adequately convey to the family or client the nature of the hearing problem and the follow-up necessary (J. McCullough, personal communication, April, 2000).

Different levels of interpreting are also noted in the courtroom. In the formal style, advanced planning of the speakers' presentations is necessary. In the consultative style, the conversation is unplanned and contains contractions, fillers, and the expression of individual background and needs. In the casual style, there is a frequent use of colloquialisms (Fowler, 1997). Even though the need for differing interpreting styles may not be directly applicable in the field of speech-language pathology and audiology, it may be helpful in situations where the interpreter needs to participate in a fair hearing or due process proceeding. Therefore, knowing the context in which an interpretation takes place and preparing adequately are critical.

> [K]nowing the context in which an interpretation takes place and preparing adequately are critical.

The interpretation process is further complicated because the context of what is translated may be totally foreign to one of the parties. For example, in the United States, rights must be disclosed to individuals before they sign a contract or agree to a procedure; this is unknown to many people from other countries. Informing someone of his or her rights is done in educational and medical contexts. Some cultures exclude the person who will receive a given medical procedure from giving his or her opinions and the individual's family takes charge (Lustig and Koester, 1999).

ANSWERS TO COMMON QUESTIONS

Here are some suggested answers to questions that may be posed to speech-language pathologists and audiologists as they interact with populations of different ages who have diverse linguistic and cultural backgrounds. Many of the questions have been posed to either one or both authors in the course of their work with multilingual and multicultural families.

Question 1: A parent of Hispanic origin asks: "Could my child's language-learning difficulty or disability have been caused by something like evil-eye or fright (*susto*) during my pregnancy?"

Answer: Listen carefully to the parent's concern and state that it might be difficult to know the source of the child's problem. Avoid making a judgment about the parent's comment. If the parent seeks a medically based explanation for a concern, it is best to refer the parent to a physician. Focus on what can be done therapeutically and educationally for the child's disability.

Question 2: "I am currently seeing a healer. Can my child's problem be cured?"

Answer: Accept what the parent says and state that you respect the parent's visit to the healer. However, it is important to clearly describe the disability to the parent and lay out paths for intervention.

Question 3: An Arabic-, Cantonese-, or Mandarin-speaking parent asks: "What do you mean when you say my child is disabled?"

Answer: The Arabic-speaking community is mostly Islamic. Its members may need a less medically based explanation for the cause of a disability because they may rely on a religiously based explanation. An explanation supported with facts might be important in helping them see the need for treatment. Cantonese and Mandarin speakers, on the other hand, may not be closely tied to any religion and are less likely to be concerned about the religious underpinnings. In either case, the focus of discussion should be on the child and the potential for improvement and progress.

Question 4: "I firmly believe that my child's language-learning difficulty is caused by her simultaneous exposure to English and Spanish. Bilingualism is very confusing to her. Why are you telling me that the problem is language based?"

Answer: If the collaborative team feels the problem is language-based and bilingualism is not directly related to the student's problems, the team must clearly explain to the parent that bilingualism by itself does not cause a disability. Provide examples of other siblings or children who are growing up bilingually and are not experiencing the same type of problem that this child is facing. The concept is sometimes difficult to convey to parents and may need to be explained over time.

Question 5: "I have no time to come to therapy. Besides, can I help if I don't speak English?

Answer: It may take several sessions and attempts before the parent realizes that his or her contributions may benefit the child. In many cases, patience may be necessary. In many cultures, the professional is believed to be the only one who can make a difference in a child. To succeed, the communication disorders professional should involve the interpreter in the process of encouraging the parent to value his or her participation in the sessions.

Question 6: "I am unable to read to my child. I don't speak English and my ability to read in my language is limited due to lack of formal education. What can I do to help my child?"

Answer: Alternatives may be suggested, such as encouraging the parent to talk to the child about the family's activities, to make up stories, to look at picture books together, or to watch TV programs as a family and discuss the content.

Question 7: "I have missed many appointments because I do not see any progress. I would rather see my husband [a stroke patient] relaxing at home instead of having to keep these appointments. Why should we keep coming?"

Answer: It might be necessary to stress the importance of consistent visits and indicate that results may not always be apparent immediately. Some patients may only improve after several months of therapy. Provide the family member with frequent feedback on the patient's progress, or involve the family member in observing and charting the progress herself.

Question 8: The husband of a patient who had a stroke is speaking to the speech-language pathologist and the dietitian at a hospital: "My wife cannot eat the foods you are serving. Our religion does not permit it. What can I do?"

Answer: The therapist and dietitian must devise a series of foods that have the necessary consistency but are also acceptable to the patient.

Question 9: "I don't see any improvement in my child's hearing when she wears her hearing aids. She did well without them the first two years of her life. Why does she need them now?"

Answer: The audiologist may emphasize that wearing the hearing aids will help the child continue to develop her language skills in the native language and also assist in a more successful transition in learning English.

Question 10: "What type of classroom would you recommend for my child who has a language lag in Spanish? How will she learn English eventually? It is so important to me that she be fluent in English but also be able to communicate with me and my family in Spanish."

Answer: Provide optimal language-learning environments using culturally sensitive approaches. When teaching is accomplished in a relevant context, the learner is able to understand and assimilate the information more thoroughly. Parental participation is strongly advocated in all instances. Specific references to successful approaches can be found in August and Hakuta (1998), and in Gersten and Jiménez (1998).

Question 11: "I don't speak English well. What language are you going to use for your therapy with my preschool child?"

Answer: This question needs to be answered pragmatically. We need to be honest about the availability of well-trained staff in the student's native language. It is best if the child receives intervention in the primary language (Kiernan and Swisher, 1990; Perozzi and Sánchez, 1992) but if this is impossible, English is acceptable. However, conscious effort should be made to encourage continuation of the primary language at home by offering specific instructions on how to stimulate the language. Staff should be sensitive to cultural issues.

Question 12: A parent asks the interpreter, "The audiologist said our child should wear the hearing aid at home and at school, but we think he should keep it at school. What do you think?"

Answer: It is common for a parents, family members, or clients to seek the advice of the interpreter because the interpreter is often the only person who can successfully communicate with the them. The interpreter's role is to provide a bridge between two individuals who cannot communicate directly because they do not share the same language. Interpreters should not provide any advice or ideas that transcend their role, and should instead refer these questions to the specialist. Speech-language pathologists and audiologists should be sure to clarify the interpreter's role ahead of time and request that interpreters refer these kinds of questions to them.

4 Assessing Culturally/Linguistically Diverse (CLD) Populations

I wanted to capture what language ability tests can never reveal: her intent, her passion, her imagery, the rhythm of her speech and the nature of her thoughts.

—*Amy Tan*

Chapter Goals

- Describe the inadequacy and limitations of standardized tests

- Discuss the influence of culture in conducting bilingual assessments

- Discuss the limited number of non-English tests and describe some

- Address the areas in which interpreters and translators must exercise caution when using formal tests, including words, structures, intonation, and discourse

- Provide a list of factors to consider prior to assessment

- Suggest a general approach to follow when conducting assessments

- Describe assessment when there are no tests in the primary language

DISCUSSION ITEMS

1. A speech-language pathologist had an English version of a standardized test translated into Bengali, and an experienced interpreter presented the test under the clinician's direction. Why would the score from this test be invalid? What would be the implications of reporting this test score?

2. What are the benefits of using formal and informal sources of information to evaluate a culturally/linguistically diverse (CLD) client?

3. If using non-English test materials, what should you keep in mind regarding norming?

4. Identify three jargon words or phrases used in your work or educational setting that would be difficult to translate into another language. How would you paraphrase a statement to facilitate the translation of these words or phrases?

5. What do you think an interpreter should do if a communication disorders professional makes a statement that seems socially inappropriate to members of the other culture?

6. What do you feel are the three most important factors to consider before assessment?

7. Identify benefits of the interpreter's participation in each step of the RIOT process.

8. Why might a speech-language pathologist ask an interpreter to readminister translated test items that the client failed on an English version of a test?

9. Role-play administering an audiological procedure to a client that does not speak English.

PITFALLS OF STANDARDIZED TESTS

For decades, communication disorders professionals have been struggling to find appropriate procedures to provide fair and appropriate assessments of culturally/linguistically diverse (CLD) populations. Interpretation and translation are integral components of such clinical encounters. Skills such as vocabulary knowledge and the ability to understand and use linguistic concepts have been the basis of many language assessments, and these are highly dependent on accurate interpreting and translating.

Researchers and scholars in speech-language pathology and psychology have written about some of the limitations and pitfalls of translations of tests. However, clinicians continue to use them almost exclusively, with limited or no reference to any other information concerning the student (Cheng, 1996; Damico, 1991; Kayser, 1995; Langdon, 1992; McGowan, Johnson, and Maxwell, 1981; Valdés and Figueroa, 1995; Valencia and Rankin, 1985). Furthermore, audiologists have used translated versions of speech-discrimination tests that have proved to be ineffective when the phonological properties of the two languages are dissimilar (J. Lang, personal communication, January 2000; J. McCullough, personal communication, April 2000).

Federal law (IDEA, 1997) specifies that an individual who needs to be assessed for special education must be evaluated in the primary language "unless it is clearly not feasible to do so," and the selection and administration of tests are not discriminatory on a racial or cultural basis (614 [b] [3] [a]). Therefore, in the absence of a bilingual clinician, it is essential that communication disorders professionals be trained to work with interpreters.

Unavailability and Inadequacy of Norms for the Primary Language

There is a great paucity of testing materials in languages other than English that provide specific information on the speech, language, and communication skills that are typically evaluated by speech-language pathologists and audiologists. Even the results of those tests that are available in Spanish need to be interpreted with care because few have been appropriately normed. Therefore, alternative measures must be devised to evaluate client's skills in their primary language.

In no case should normed tests be translated into the other language for any purpose other than simply observing a client's performance (i.e., not to obtain a score). The level of difficulty of a given item is most often not equivalent across languages, so norms cannot be used because they have not been developed for the second language. Even when norms have been established for a given language, they may not be entirely applicable to a particular client. Dialectal differences impact meaning and are common in many languages. In addition, each client has had very specific exposure to each language, which influences his or her linguistic and communicative competence. Consequently, tests provide only a partial view of any client's linguistic and communicative competence.

Translating tests from one language to another has been a frequently used strategy by clinicians to evaluate linguistic skills in a client's primary language. The entire assessment is complicated because test results must be deciphered based on stages in linguistic acquisition, which vary from language to language and culture to culture. A good example of the variation in developmental sequence occurs for quantifiers in Chinese. These words are complex and have no counterparts in most other languages. Yet, the degree of sophistication of these quantifiers can be used to measure language development in Chinese children. Additionally, the length of individual words is sometimes used as a yardstick for English language development. In contrast, Cantonese Chinese is essentially monosyllabic, so length does not play such an important role in the assessment of this language. Word length is not equivalent between languages, either. A

> [L]ength needs to be considered when translating or adapting any material because it may influence memory and expression.

Spanish language version, for example, might be slightly longer than an English version. Many common words such as *zapato* (shoe), *abrigo* (coat), *pantalón* (pants), and *manzana* (apple) are longer in Spanish than their English counterparts. Therefore, length needs to be considered when translating or adapting any material because it may influence memory and expression. Frequency of occurrence of words in one language may also differ significantly between languages, so tests based on frequency of occurrence are not directly translatable.

Cross-linguistic and cross-cultural research data indicate many differences in language acquisition. For example, Choi (1997) reported that unlike English speakers, Korean-speaking and Mandarin-speaking children learn verbs and nouns in a parallel manner. The generally accepted view that children all over the world develop nouns first may therefore need to be reexamined and challenged. The clinical implications of such cross-linguistic research are significant in guiding the translation of tests from one language to another and for deciphering test results based on language-specific normative data and input.

Disregard for Unique Cultural, Linguistic, and Experiential Backgrounds

Traditionally, communication disorders professionals working with the CLD population may not have been trained in or considered the influence of this population's cultural and experiential background on its responses to testing and evaluation. Many diagnoses have been made following the results of standardized tests, which were based on the mainstream monolingual English population. Added to the cultural variations are the ways questions are posed, including the media in which test items are presented. There are also item types and formats that clients have never encountered. Input from significant others, teachers, or other staff working with CLD individuals has not been considered on a consistent basis in the evaluation or diagnosis of a possible language or learning disability.

In the last 30 years or so, with the advent of federal special education legislation, changes have been noted in the process of assessing the CLD population. Special educators have more often taken into account the unique cultural, linguistic, and experiential backgrounds of CLD students. The requirement to assess students in the language they normally use has resulted in more appropriate assessment procedures. As a result of this legislation, norms have been used only when appropriate for a given individual. Thus, caution has been taken to evaluate the individual based on performance on informal as well as formal tests, portfolios, observations, and progress over time. Resources such as Goldstein (2000), Langdon and Saenz (1996), and Roseberry-McKibbin (1995) offer several suggestions on how to collect and integrate additional information in the process of evaluating CLD students. These procedures can also be applied to older clients. The traditional focus for assessment, which did not take cultural factors into account, is contrasted with the preferred focus in assessing students who are CLD in Table 4.1 (see page 68).

Limited Availability of Non-English Test Materials

Several tests are currently available in Spanish, but there are virtually no tests that have been developed in other languages, except for the Bilingual Verbal Ability Test (BVAT) (Muñoz-Sandoval, Cummins, Alvarado, and Ruef, 1998). This test assesses a number of languages including Arabic, Chinese, French, German, Haitian-Creole, Hindi, Italian, Japanese,

Table 4.1 Traditional vs. Preferred Focus for Assessment

Traditional Focus	Preferred Focus
Assessment personnel unfamiliar with the CLD population	Assessment personnel familiar with the language and culture of the CLD population
Family and health information collected in English without assistance from an interpreter	Family and health information collected with assistance from an interpreter to evaluate the client's language and cultural background
Testing in English only	Testing in English and the primary language (when appropriate)
Use of standardized procedures	Use of multiple sources of information, such as questionnaires, portfolios, and language samples
Norms based on U.S. population	Norms used only when appropriate
Input from other professionals and family not considered in decision making regarding eligibility	Input from other professionals and family considered in decision making regarding eligibility

Source: Ortiz, García, and Wilkinson (1988)

Korean, Polish, Portuguese, Russian, Spanish, Turkish, and Vietnamese. Only receptive and expressive vocabulary knowledge and word associations are assessed.

A limited number of tests have been normed on bilingual Spanish-English speaking students, including the Spanish edition of the Clinical Evaluation of Language Fundamentals–3 (CELF–3) (Wiig, Secord, and Semel, 1997) and the Pruebas de Expresión Oral y Percepción de la Lengua Española (PEOPLE) (Mares, 1980). A few others, such as the Test de Vocabulario en Imágenes Peabody (TVIP) (Dunn, Padilla, Lugo, and Dunn, 1986) and the Spanish version of the Woodcock Language

Proficiency Battery–Revised (WLPB–R) (Woodcock, 1981), have been normed on various groups of monolingual Spanish-speaking subjects. When these tests are used, speech-language pathologists and audiologists must use the normative data with caution because the norming samples had specific characteristics that may not match those of the individual being assessed.

Tests for children that have been normed in Spanish include the Batería de Lenguaje Objectivo y Criterial (BLOC) (Puyuelo, Wiig, Renom, and Solanas, 1998), Cuaderno de Logoaudiometría (audiometric notebook) (Cárdenas and Marrero, 1994), and Protocolo para la Valoración de la Audición y el Lenguaje en Lengua Española en un Programa de Implantes Cocleares (a protocol to measure hearing and speech in Spanish speakers who have cochlear implants) (Huarte, Molina, Manrique, Olleta, and García-Tapia, 1996).

Other tests have been adapted or translated into Spanish, but they have not been normed on native speakers or bilingual individuals, for example, the Preschool Language Scale–3 (PLS–3), Spanish version (Zimmerman, Steiner, and Pond, 1993). The Spanish edition of the Boston Diagnostic Aphasia Examination (Revised) (Goodglass and Kaplan, 1983) was translated and adapted by García-Albea, Sánchez, and Del Viso (1982) from an earlier version of the test. Tests developed and normed in other languages are emerging, including the Arabic Language Screening Tests: Preschool and School-Age (El-Halees and Wiig, 1999) and the Arabic Receptive-Expressive Vocabulary Test (El-Halees and Wiig, 2000), which have been normed in Jordan and Palestine. Appendix B includes available tests that have been normed, translated, or adapted into Spanish or other languages for various ages.

Because of their limitations and the lack of tests in languages other than English, speech-language pathologists or audiologists must use other procedures to arrive at correct diagnoses. The scope of this chapter does not permit an extensive discussion regarding best practices in assessing the speech, language, and communication skills of CLD clients. Speech-language pathologists and audiologists are referred to sources such as Battle (1993); Cheng (1991); Kayser (1995, 1998); Langdon (1992b); and a reference written in Spanish by Puyuelo, Rondal, and Wiig (2000). All these authors recommend collecting information from a variety of sources, such as the family, the teachers, and the client, to arrive at a correct diagnosis. Tests should be only one component of assessment. Other components may include a language sample, responses to questionnaires, observations, reading and writing samples from the client in the primary language (if the client has been exposed to written language), and evaluations of portfolios.

CHALLENGES OF FORMAL TESTS

Words

Four types of challenges exist when attempting to interpret or translate words from one language to another:

1. A given word often does not have a single counterpart word in another language. For example:

   - The recommended Hmong translation for *parasite* requires 24 words, *hormone* requires 31 words, and *X chromosome* requires 46 words (Fadiman, 1997).

- Several words are needed to define the Swahili word *pole* (po'-leh), and still the full meaning might not be entirely conveyed. *Pole* is a comment used when a person experiences something unfortunate, from a simple misstep to something as tragic as the death of a loved one. If the person stumbles, the word means *poor you*, or *too bad*. The word can also be used to imply *I am sorry, I sympathize and hope you get well soon, I offer you my condolences, I am sorry to hear the person died*, or *I sympathize and hope you will be OK*. (O. K. Ogwaro, personal communication, May, 1997).

2. One word may designate several items in another language. For example:

- The word that means *bread* in Chinese may mean *bagel, croissant, roll*, or *toast*. The Chinese *yu* can mean *shower, downpour*, or *drizzle* in English.

- In Vietnamese, the word for *hair* also means *feather*. The Chinese word for *challenge (zan)*, literally translated as *pick a fight*, connotes aggression and a warlike attitude, and the word for *propaganda (tung zan)*, literally translated as *general fight*, also contains the word *zan*, connoting a war-like attitude.

- Some prepositions differ from language to language. *Kiita* in Korean means both *in* and *on* in English (Choi, 1997; Gopnick and Choi, 1995). The same goes for other languages (e.g., the Spanish word *adentro* can mean *in* and *inside*). In some languages, inflection within words may designate the position of the

71

object. Thus, a test that assesses prepositions may become a test that assesses inflections instead.

3. Words carry a different meaning in different cultures, even within the same language. For example:

- Inviting someone to tea in Australia means being invited to dinner, while inviting someone to tea in the United Stated means to have a cup of tea.

- In England, the word *bathroom* implies a room with a bathtub in it, while in the United States, it means a room with a toilet in it.

- In African American English, *brim* means *hat*, *knuckles* means *gloves*, and *glass house* implies *jail*. *Girlfriend* connotes intimacy and the words *main squeeze* are used to mean boyfriend.

4. Some words cannot be translated, because no equivalent exists in the other language and the words are very culturally bound or culturally specific. For example:

- *Bar mitzva* is Hebrew for the reaching of adult responsibilities for a Jewish boy and the celebration marking the occasion.

- *Curandero* means something similar to a spiritual healer in Mexico.

- *Quinceañera* in Spanish represents a Latin American girl turning fifteen, somewhat equivalent to the North American sweet sixteen.

- *Gemutlich* is German for something similar to *cozy*.

- The English word *background* has very few exact equivalents in other languages.

In summary, even single words are difficult to interpret or translate from one language to another. Furthermore, there may be different gradations of difficulty. For example, in written language, the number of strokes in a Chinese dialect may determine the difficulty of the character, while in English the difficulty of a word is influenced by the number of syllables and the frequency of occurrence.

Word meanings provided by a dictionary may not convey current or extended meanings or, very importantly, connotations. Individuals who are familiar with local meanings may need to be consulted to get to the true meaning of a given word.

> **Word meanings provided by a dictionary may not convey current or extended meanings or, very importantly, connotations.**

To make translations culturally fair and linguistically appropriate, clinicians have suggested the process of back-translation. In *back translation*, the translated word is retranslated into the original language to ensure accuracy and matching of meanings. Challenges like these occur frequently in the daily practice of many speech-language pathologists and audiologists. To illustrate, E. Li (personal communication, July 7, 1997) described a research project on translation in which a group of 20 Chinese-English bilingual and biliterate individuals were asked to translate a list of single English words into Chinese. Results indicated that several of the words were translated in many different ways, for example:

- The word *fall* was translated as leaves *fall, fall because of tripping, fall because one is not steady, fall from a high place, drop, raindrops, you fall because someone pushes you,* and *the fall season.*

- The word *frightened* was translated using various words in Chinese, including *fear, fright, scared, scared to death, fearful, horrified, terrified, afraid,* and *frightened.*

- The word *sad* was translated using several different words in Chinese, including *upset, disappointed, melancholic, sad, heartbroken, hurt, worried, worrisome, grieved,* and *unhappy.*

- The word *make* was translated as *produce, make, manufacture, design, do,* and *fabricate.*

The Chinese translators who were attempting to translate the words from English into Chinese found it difficult to locate a cultural and linguistic fit for these words without knowing the context. Thus, for example, in developing an augmentative communication device to be used in both Chinese and English, the following strategies were suggested for use by speech-language pathologists and audiologists: (1) choose the name that the greatest number of Chinese people use through consensus, (2) choose the one with the same number of syllables, (3) drop the item if an appropriate counterpart cannot be found, (4) use all the Chinese words and have them translated into English through back translation, (5) have a larger group of bilingual-biliterate individuals do the same translation and provide back translation to reach a consensus, and (6) define the word with a context so that words with multiple meanings can be interpreted appropriately.

Structures

An interpreter or translator must know and understand the structure of the two languages because a word-by-word interpretation or translation results in an inaccurate transmission of meaning or incorrect structure in the second language. Variations may exist across languages and within dialects. For example:

- The German phrase "Den Junge hat der Hund gebissen" is literally interpreted as "The boy has the dog bit." The object-verb-subject word order is allowable in German but is incorrect if used in English. The correct English interpretation would be, "The dog bit the boy."

- In some languages, like French, the subject-verb order is maintained, just as in English. But, a negation is expressed with two morphemes, one at each side of the verb (e.g., *je comprend* [I understand] becomes *je ne comprend pas* [I do not understand]).

- A phrase that means "you go first" is interpreted following the English order in Cantonese, but not in Mandarin, where it is interpreted as "you first go."

- Idioms and metaphors can be meaningless in other languages. For example, *a piece of cake,* meaning *easy,* cannot be translated in another language word by word. *Pie in the sky* is not used in any other language.

Speech-language pathologists and audiologists should limit their use of idioms and metaphors during interactions requiring an interpreter or translator. Communication disorders professionals should be aware of the structural differences between languages. If a client uses non-English grammatical structures, these professionals should confer with the interpreter or translator and determine if the structure is that of the primary language.

Intonation

Intonation (i.e., change of pitch, stress, or juncture) plays an important role in the meaning of a phrase or sentence, and it must be considered for accurate interpreting. The question "How are you?" has a different intonation when used to greet someone as contrasted with a nurse or doctor checking on a patient. In many Asian languages, tones play a crucial role in conveying meaning, and the interpreter must pay close attention to these features. As Hermes (1998) indicated, there are few rules to guide nonnative listeners. A change of tone is not particular to Asian languages only, but may occur in Spanish, Norwegian, and English (Flege and Bohn, 1989). For example, the phrase "I did produce" with the stress on the second syllable of *produce* means something different than when the stress is on the first syllable. A different stress on each of the two syllables in the word *compound* implies either a chemical or adding on to something. In Spanish, there is a difference between "¿cómo está?" (How are you?) and "como esta" (I eat this one or like this one, depending on the context). A well-known example of intonation and its effect in English is "I saw the white *house*" and "I saw the *White* House." In some West African languages, like Twi or Akan spoken in Ghana, the change of tone refers to a different verb tense. Other examples that focus on the importance of intonation can be found in Campbell (1995), Cheng (1996, 1998b), and Crystal (1997).

Discourse

Discourse refers to the structure of a language used in situations such as a conversation, an interview, a speech, a learning situation, or a testing environment. Certain rules need to be followed in these contexts to initiate and end the interaction and to collaborate among the parties involved to achieve successful communication.

At times, successful communication between speakers who do not share the same language may be complicated because of different expectations regarding rules and the definition of "safe" topics. For example, in some cultures, one does not discuss personal information. Therefore, asking questions about a mother's pregnancy and delivery may not be appropriate in an educational setting and should be reserved for a physician or nurse interview only.

> [S]uccessful communication between speakers who do not share the same language may be complicated because of different expectations.

The manner in which questions are posed is also important. It is difficult to define what is polite, proper, or improper because there are cross-cultural variations. Also, as stated in Chapter 3, parents who are asked to be partners in the assessment and intervention process may have differing views about their role in the process because special education is a new concept for them and they believe that the communication disorders professional is the authority.

The success of a conversation may differ because some cultures take a circular route rather than a linear/sequential route in transmitting information. Therefore, making culturally and linguistically appropriate interpretations requires high-level metalinguistic abilities and cross-cultural competence.

Resources for Cultural Competency

Information on families of Asian/Pacific Island origin:
Cheng, L.L. (1998). Beyond multiculturalism: Cultural translators make it happen. In V.O. Pang and L.L. Cheng (Eds.), *Struggling to be heard* (pp. 105–122). Albany, NY: SUNY Press.

Information on families of Hispanic origin:
Harry, B. (1992). *Cultural diversity, families and the special education system.* New York: Teachers College Press.

Information on 177 countries and cultural practices:
CultureGrams (www.CultureGrams.com)

Information on learning English in children and adults:
Center for Applied Linguistics (www.cal.org)

Information on second language learning and culturally responsive pedagogy:
Diaz-Rico, L.T., and Weed, K.A. (1995). *The crosscultural, language, and academic development handbook: A complete K–12 reference guide.* Boston: Allyn and Bacon.

Cultural differences are evident in children's behavior and response in a learning environment. Cheng (1991) provided a list of considerations that speech-language pathologists, audiologists, and interpreters should take into account when observing a student in a classroom setting. For example, students may not ask or respond to questions because of teacher respect. In other cultures, students do not challenge the teacher, they help one another, they stay at their desk and do not wander in the room, and they do not expect parents to know what teachers know. Cultural differences that apply to Hispanic and other populations are discussed in Harry (1992); Lynch and Hanson (1992); and Pedersen, Draguns, Lonner, and Trimble (1996).

Communication disorders professionals' discourse rules also vary depending on their background and expectations. For example, one research study found that CLD students may be asked to respond less frequently, and that their responses may go unrecognized more often than those of Anglo students (Schinke-Llano, 1983). Furthermore, Kayser (1995) found that Spanish-speaking clinicians used more touching to get a child's attention as compared to English-speaking clinicians when the parties were engaged in a testing situation. Communication disorders professionals should keep in mind, however, that individual differences must be considered regardless of reported observations for designated groups.

ASSESSMENT
WITH AN INTERPRETER

General Preassessment Guidelines

Before conducting an assessment or deciding that an interpreter is needed, the communication disorders professional and the assessment team must consider the following eight factors:

1. *Personal factors*: Attitude, motivation, and anxiety influence the speed at which individuals learn a second language (Mitchell and Myles, 1998). Some students are less self-conscious or more confident than others and, therefore, have less difficulty acquiring a second language. They approach native speakers more readily and engage in conversation, which enables them to use and expand their proficiency in the second language (Wong-Fillmore, 1991).

2. *Adjustment issues:* Some immigrants experience cultural discontinuities, and others adjust very quickly and very well. Historical, sociological, and political components in immigrants' adjustments to a new environment need to be considered (Suárez-Orozco, 1989; Trueba, Cheng, and Ima, 1993; Trueba, Jacobs, and Kirton, 1990).

3. *Use of each language:* English may be the language used at school or at work only, and the student, therefore, may have limited exposure to the English language at home. Furthermore, the use of each language is different depending on the context. Cummins (1984) differentiates

two levels of language proficiency. Basic Interpersonal Communication Skills (BICS) is the type of language used when an individual's communication is enhanced by context (e.g., when the communication relates to an experience or during a face-to-face communication). On the other hand, Cognitive Academic Language Proficiency (CALP) refers to a more abstract level of communication that is needed to succeed in school. At this level, the second language learner acquires information from situations that are more decontextualized,

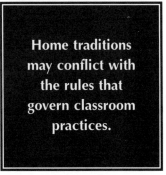

Home traditions may conflict with the rules that govern classroom practices.

(e.g., reading and lectures) and communicates about events that are more abstract (e.g., science concepts).

4. *Type of discourse:* CLD students often experience what Cheng (1994a) called "difficult discourse" due to socio-logical and psychological difficulties that arise when adaptation to a different or dual culture and language is necessary. Home traditions may conflict with the rules that govern classroom practices. Although stereotypes should be avoided, having a general knowledge about how various groups adapt to a new linguistic environment is helpful to understand why some groups may have more difficulty than others. For example, Chinese, Japanese, and Korean families often empha-size literacy and are motivated to learn English.

On the other hand, Lao, Khmer, and Hmong families come from more traditional agricultural backgrounds where formal education may not have been emphasized, so families may be not as motivated to learn English (Cheng, 1994a).

5. *Home-school differences:* Many CLD students from Hispanic or Asian backgrounds may be hesitant when participating in class (Cheng, 1994a; Langdon and Clark, 1993). For example, "in traditional Hispanic/Latino cultures, children are taught to listen, to obey, and not to challenge older persons or persons of authority, such as parents or teachers" (Langdon and Clark, 1993, p. 96).

6. *Learning styles:* Some students study alone, others in groups. Some study in quiet environments, others thrive amidst distractions (García, 1991; Tharp and Gallimore, 1991).

7. *Nonverbal cues:* Eye gaze, physical contact, and body language influence communication, and cultures differ in ways in which communication is nonverbally transmitted and processed.

8. *Code switching and language loss:* Code switching may depend on context (Martin-Jones, 1995) and is expected in bilingual communication (Langdon and Merino, 1992). Questions about expressive language must take into account the natural loss of a language that is infrequently used.

RIOT: A Suggested Procedure for Assessment

The review, interview, observe, and test (RIOT) procedure has been found effective in identifying factors that may prevent CLD students from succeeding in school or other learning environments while ensuring that inappropriate special education referrals and placements are not carried out (Leung, 1995). RIOT can also be applied in the assessment of adults. (See Appendix C for a case study.) The steps in the RIOT procedure are:

1. *Review* the following pieces of information: school and medical records; reports; teachers' comments; linguistic, cultural, social, and family background; and previous therapy or testing results.

2. *Interview* teachers, peers, family members, and other informants. Questionnaires are available from multiple sources to obtain all the necessary information (Cheng, 1990, 1991, 1995; Langdon, 1992b; Westby, 1990). It is very important to include the family's or parents' perceptions of their child's skills or aptitudes as well as areas of difficulty. Often, results of a thorough interview assist the team in planning the assessment process. For example, finding out that a student had difficulties learning the primary language or has had a significant medical history assists in determining that the student is experiencing a language-learning difficulty rather than a language difference. Also, if the parent reports that the student has had limited exposure to school and literacy

activities, it indicates that the student may need more time to acquire skills prior to being assessed. In addition, finding out the level of literacy that an individual had prior to a traumatic injury assists in determining loss of skills resulting from the injury.

The speech-language pathologist and audiologist may interview the parents or family to gain information about play activities, what the student likes to do at home, the student's play and interaction partners in the home setting, any major event in the student's life that may compound the problem, and how the parents and family have reacted to the student's language performance. These important pieces of information will provide a more complete picture of the student outside the school. A teacher interview should also be conducted to find out the student's ability to follow oral and written directions in the classroom, his or her progress over time, response to various types of accommodations, and a comparison of the student with others who have similar linguistic and scholastic experiences.

3. *Observe* a student in multiple contexts with a variety of people. Observations of the student's interactions at school (inside and outside the classroom context) and at home assist in gaining a broader picture of the student's language dominance and preference. In addition, observations enable the assessment team to define contexts that are conducive to more successful learning. The interpreter can assist in providing additional input on the student's behavior and language and compare the

student with peers with similar dual linguistic and environmental backgrounds. In health-care settings, observing the client communicating with familiar and unfamiliar people enables the speech-language pathologist to form a broader perspective of the client's skills. A more comprehensive understanding of a client's daily activities enables the audiologist to provide a more appropriate hearing device.

> **Analyzing the student's portfolio assists in gaining a better understanding about how the student has progressed over time.**

4. *Test* school/work and home language competence using multiple sources of information, such as informal assessments, language samples, and specific test materials (if available in a given language and being cautious about norming procedures). The evaluation may be supported by further use of authentic and dynamic assessment procedures. Analyzing the student's portfolio assists in gaining a better understanding about how the student has progressed over time.

The nature of collaboration with the interpreter will be different in each situation. When collecting a more comprehensive health and developmental history from the parent or family, the interpreter will need to utilize interviewing skills. At other times, the interpreter may observe the student in various environments or assist the speech-language pathologist in assessing the language. The interpreter should not be left alone during an assessment or during an intervention session, even if the interpreter has had experience administering and recording responses to a given set of instruments. Taping the entire assessment process enables the speech-language pathologist and the interpreter to review any segment of the interaction and to transcribe the student's responses or language sample.

Speech-Language Assessment When There Are No Tests in the Primary Language

Because there are so few tests that have been adequately translated or normed, speech-language pathologists may need to collaborate with interpreters to use other sources of information that provide a clearer picture of a client's communication ability. Two main options exist:

1. Administer a given test in English first, even if a client has limited skills, unless his or her skills are so limited that the experience might be counterproductive. Readminister the failed items in the client's primary language by using a careful translation of those items. However, extreme caution needs to be exercised so that the level of difficulty is equivalent in both languages. Some words translate with lexicon that is generally easier (e.g., *compel* is translated to Polish with the word *zmuszac,* which is more commonly used and heard than the English *compel*). Other words may have two possible translations, like *gigantic,* which can translate to Polish

as *gigantyczny* or *kolosalny*. In no instance should norms be calculated on this translated test, because the results would violate principles of validity and reliability.

2. Supplement the test information by using various functional questionnaires and interest finders and by obtaining a language sample in a client's primary language. Document responses to various types of questions and situations. The interpreter must be specifically trained on how to elicit a language sample. It is best if the sample is recorded and subsequently transcribed. Depending on the client's age, the sample may be obtained from informal conversations, describing a personal experience, retelling a story or a movie, formulating a story from a comic strip or a wordless book, or responding to a set of questions or comments that elicit an opinion on a particular subject. The analysis of the sample should include assessment of phonology, semantics, syntax, formulation skills, ability to respond to questions and comments, organization of a narrative, and analysis of various communicative functions.

Audiological Assessment When There Are No Tests in the Primary Language

Due to a lack of literature on this subject, the following description of the interpreting process is based on an oral interview with J. McCullough (personal communication, April 13, 2000), an audiologist and university professor. Although the views reported may not be practiced by all audiologists who work with CLD clients, it is considered fairly typical.

Because there is such a paucity of phonetically balanced word lists in languages other than Spanish and Vietnamese, the audiologist's testing battery is often limited to pure-tone testing and general speech-threshold awareness. However, new lists for various languages are being developed.

Most commonly, a client sees an audiologist to evaluate the presence and degree of a hearing loss. The procedure includes pure-tone testing and speech discrimination. In addition, the client may receive a tympanogram to assess middle ear function. Even when the client has minimal or no understanding of English, showing and asking which ear might have a problem or whether the client experiences dizziness or ringing in the ear can be demonstrated with gestures. McCullough reported that in her practice, 80% of her patients speak a language other

> **Because of the objectivity of a typical audiological evaluation, the need for an interpreter is not as crucial.**

than English, most typically Vietnamese, Mandarin, or Spanish. She is able to convey information and the client responds adequately using a nonverbal mode of communication. Because of the objectivity of a typical audiological evaluation, the need for an interpreter is not as crucial. However, the participation of an interpreter in aural rehabilitation is important. However, because the different hearing aids and their uses can be demonstrated and seen, a person performing the duties of an interpreter does not need to know much about technological terms, but accuracy of interpretation continues to be very important. Many of the qualities and skills that an interpreter should possess are still applicable when collaborating with an audiologist. The interpreter should be someone who is fluent in the two languages, remains neutral, respects confidentiality, is empathetic, and likes to interact with people from various walks of life. An additional quality is that the interpreter who works with hearing impaired patients should speak clearly and loudly, but with moderation (J. McCullough, personal communication, April 13, 2000).

One of the drawbacks of assessing patients who speak a different language is the inability to check the results of the pure-tone testing with speech-discrimination testing. It is inappropriate to ask clients to repeat English words because their knowledge of the language may be limited. On the other hand, asking clients to repeat words in their own language from a tape does not yield accurate results, because the audiologist who does not speak the client's language cannot evaluate the accuracy of the client's response.

McCullough has worked on procedures to develop phonetically balanced lists in other languages, including Russian, Mandarin, and Vietnamese. However, specialized equipment is necessary and the technology is not yet readily available that would provide an audiologist with the needed feedback regarding the client's ability to discriminate words in the primary language by matching the client's production to the target word. In preliminary trials, the client is asked to point to one of four pictured words that vary slightly from one another, such as _nol_ (zero), _nosh_ (knife), _nos_ (nose), and _notch_ (night) (Aleksandrovsky, McCullough, and Wilson,

1998; McCullough, Wilson, Birck, and Anderson, 1994). In the near future, with the advances of voice recognition, McCullough predicts that computers will be able to evaluate the accuracy of the client's word repetitions.

5 Interpreting and Translating in Speech-Language Pathology and Audiology

The responsibility of transmitting another person's thoughts should never be taken lightly.

—*Monika Gehrke*

Chapter Goals

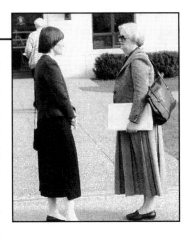

- Describe the responsibilities of a speech-language pathologist or audiologist that ensure a successful interpreting/translating process, including following a code of ethics, participating in interpreter recruitment, preparing interpreters for assignments, updating and training interpreters, understanding the interpreting process, and evaluating interpreters

- Describe the responsibilities of an interpreter or a translator that ensure a successful interpreting/translating process, including maintaining linguistic skills, following a code of ethics, maintaining neutrality and confidentiality, interpreting faithfully, engaging in ongoing learning, and remaining flexible

- Review the briefing, interaction, and debriefing (BID) process for interviews, conferences, assessments, and intervention

DISCUSSION ITEMS

1. Why is it important for communication disorders professionals to have a code of ethics for working with interpreters and translators?

2. What characteristics should a communication disorders professional look for when recruiting an interpreter?

3. Role-play assisting an interpreter to review the contents and administration of a test that will be used during an assessment.

4. What resources could the communication disorders professional call on to assist an interpreter in updating his or her skills?

5. How does understanding the interpreting process help the communication disorders professional to be more effective?

6. Why should the communication disorders professional provide input into the interpreter's performance evaluation?

7. Which of the six linguistic skills (see pages 101–102) would you consider least important when initially hiring an interpreter?

8. Role-play a meeting with an interpreter to discuss an observed deficit in one of the 11 areas listed in the interpreter's code of ethics (see page 110).

9. When should these determinations be made and who should be involved in making them?

   • Did the client understand the assessment task?

   • Should test items be repeated or rephrased?

10. Prepare a budget request for an interpreter.

SPEECH-LANGUAGE PATHOLOGIST AND AUDIOLOGIST RESPONSIBILITIES

Speech-language pathologists and audiologists who work with an interpreter have six main responsibilities:

1. Following a professional code of ethics

2. Participating in the recruitment of interpreters

3. Adequately preparing interpreters for a given assignment

4. Updating and training interpreters

5. Understanding the process of interpretation

6. Evaluating interpreter performance

Each responsibility is described in greater detail in the following sections.

Following a Professional Code of Ethics

There is no reference to working with interpreters in the ASHA (1994) Code of Ethics. The ASHA (1998) guidelines for working with interpreters, however, state that speech-language pathologists and audiologists must be trained to use interpreters effectively.

A code of ethics for speech-language pathologists and audiologists working with interpreters should emphasize the importance of following a professional protocol that protects clients and families. See the code of ethics proposed in the sidebar below. Professionals should also contribute to the knowledge base of the profession by sharing their knowledge and experience with others in the profession.

Code of Ethics for Speech-Language Pathologists and Audiologists Working with Interpreters

1. Have knowledge of bilingual language development and assessment and intervention issues.

2. Work with a trained interpreter only.

3. Continue to update knowledge through continuing education in the field of bilingualism, including assessment of and intervention with bilingual speakers.

4. Adequately prepare the interpreter for a given conference, assessment, or intervention.

5. Participate in improving the process of working with the interpreter.

6. Document successful strategies in working with the interpreter to serve bilingual clients more equitably.

Participating in the Recruitment of Interpreters

Speech-language pathologists or audiologists should be included in the process of interviewing candidates for interpreter positions since they will be working closely with these individuals. Valuable information can be obtained during an interview, such as the interpreter's level of oral and written language performance in the two languages (see "Proficiency in Two Languages," page 137), the interpreter's educational background and experiences, and a general sense of the interpreter's personal characteristics and style. For example, the candidate's responsiveness, flexibility, motivation, and willingness to learn new information can be important factors to consider. Usually, it is preferable to select a bilingual individual who has had experience working in an educational or clinical setting. The candidate may be recruited from schools, county offices of education, or service agencies. Bilingual personnel may also be recruited from community and health centers, churches, universities, community colleges, or embassies.

Speech-language pathologists or audiologists should refrain from asking for services from a bilingual individual who has not been trained to fulfill the role of an interpreter. As Pochhacker (1997) stated:

> It would be difficult even for a trained professional to interpret the native output of a dysgrammatic child in such a way as to permit a diagnostic assessment by the therapist, let alone interpretation by a close relative or a cleaning woman....Things seem to be more

fundamentally wrong, however, if a five-year-old Albanian receives his much-needed hearing aids for US$2,000 apiece but cannot receive subsequent remedial therapy because no one would think of calling in, and paying for, an interpreter. (p. 224)

In some cases, it may be impossible to find an adequately trained interpreter in a given language and, therefore, a lesser-trained person may be required to fulfill the role. It is not advisable to ask a family member, a neighbor, or a child to act as an interpreter, because these indi-

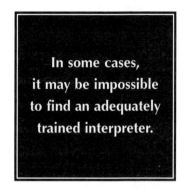

In some cases, it may be impossible to find an adequately trained interpreter.

viduals have not been adequately trained and they may not be able to remain neutral. The request is unfair to the client, the family, and the person who is asked to perform the functions of an interpreter.

Despite the inherent problems, there were situations where minors were asked to perform the role of an interpreter. In fact, their role was that of *broker* (McQuillan and Tse, 1995). "Essentially, language brokering involves interpreting and translating performed by bilinguals in daily situations without any special training" (Tse, 1995, p. 181). Brokers mediate rather than transmit communication (i.e., they typically explain the essence of a communication rather than translate the precise message). Thus, individuals utilizing the assistance of minors or untrained personnel need to understand the differences between brokering and interpreting.

Accessibility to adequately trained interpreters has been limited in some hospital settings due to lack of funding. For example, an interpreter may only be available to speak on the phone with the client and the audiologist. This practice is of limited value to either the audiologist or the client. Often, the interpreter is not adequately trained, not fully proficient in English, and does not know the nature of the given profession. Additionally, the context itself is not conducive to successful communication. The professional must be aware of the varieties in a given language spoken by the interpreter. For example, an interpreter might speak Cantonese rather than the client's Chinese dialect or may speak a specific dialect of Spanish. In these cases, the interpreter must adjust his or her vocabulary to that of the client or family. Also, a client who is hearing impaired cannot rely on facial cues from the interpreter to augment the meaning of what is happening when the interpreter speaks through a telephone. Often, the audiologist and the interpreter have never had a face-to-face meeting, so their teaming is of limited value and the quality of services is diminished (J. Lang, personal communication, April 12, 2000).

Adequately Preparing Interpreters for a Given Assignment

The speech-language pathologist or audiologist should always meet with the interpreter prior to any assignment, even though the two may have worked together in the past. The preparation might be impossible when there is an emergency and a client needs to be assessed within a short time. However, there

should be some time allotted for the speech-language pathologist or audiologist to review the background of the client and
plan the necessary steps to take in conducting an interview, a
conference, or an assessment. No meeting or encounter will
ever be completely predictable, but planning in advance assists
in coping with the unexpected more readily.

The speech-language pathologist or audiologist and the
interpreter must carefully review the directions for specific
testing before the session. They need to agree on an action plan
for how to proceed in case the client does not cooperate, has
difficulty responding to the demands of a given task, or performs better than expected. If adjustments to this plan are
needed during the course of a session, the communication disorders professional must communicate these adjustments to
the interpreter so that together they can continue an effective
collaboration.

Updating and Training Interpreters

There is great variation in interpreter training from agency to
agency. Additionally, it takes time for the speech-language
pathologist or audiologist to learn to work with an interpreter. Training is frequently offered to interpreters only, with
no involvement of the communication disorders professionals who will be working with them. However, training should
also be offered to speech-language pathologists or audiologists to ensure that the interpreting and translating process is
based on best practices. Only a few programs have reported
specific training strategies for interpreters to work with

speech-language pathologists in the educational setting (Manuel-Dupont and Yoakum, 1997; Matsuda and O'Connor, 1993). Most in-service education has been directed at interpreters only. The simultaneous training of speech-language pathologists or audiologists and interpreters has been omitted because it has been assumed that the issues pertained to the work of interpreters exclusively. Manuel-Dupont and Yoakum (1997) stated, "Further training CPs [cooperative personnel] in conjunction with IPs [interpreter professionals] and allowing time for IPs and CPs to develop and function as a team was also identified as a critical component of the IP's preparation program" (p. 95). It is essential that both parties, the speech-language pathologist or audiologist and the interpreter, learn to discuss and work together on issues that will

> It is essential that both parties, the speech-language pathologist or audiologist and the interpreter, learn to discuss and work together.

enhance the success of the process. More information on the education of speech-language pathologists and audiologists who collaborate with interpreters is provided in Chapter 6.

Understanding the Process of Interpretation

Even though the services of an interpreter are important, all parties involved must realize that the speech-language pathologist or the audiologist is ultimately the professional who is

responsible for the tone of the meeting, the diagnosis, the recommendations, the outcomes, the intervention plan, and the
follow-up. The speech-pathologist or audiologist should convey information that is clear and unambiguous. He or she must
develop a system of communication to determine when something is unclear or too lengthy to interpret during a meeting or
an assessment. Avoiding unnecessary jargon and idiomatic
expressions facilitates the interpreter's task. When the speech-
language pathologist, audiologist, or any member of a conference does not understand a certain message, it is acceptable to
request a retranslation. This strategy may not always be per-
mitted in an assessment process where specific directions must
be followed and should be explained to all participants at the
outset of a session.

Evaluating Interpreter Performance

The speech-language pathologist or audiologist must ensure
that the interpretation process is adequately followed and,
therefore, evaluation of the interpreter's ongoing performance
is necessary. The evaluator should be trained in how to work
effectively with an interpreter and be knowledgeable about the
roles and responsibilities of interpreters. If an administrator
other than the speech-language pathologist or audiologist is
responsible for performing staff evaluations, the administrator
should seek input from the communication disorders professional. Input should also be gathered from consumers of the
interpreter services. Evaluation is described in greater detail in
Chapter 6 (see "On-the-Job Evaluation," page 146).

INTERPRETER AND TRANSLATOR RESPONSIBILITIES

As was stated in previous chapters, the interpreter's or translator's responsibility is to bridge communication in various contexts between parties who do not share the same language. In the practice of speech-language pathology and audiology, these contexts include interviews and conferences with parents or family members, testing and assessment, intervention, and due process hearings. Each one of these contexts requires knowledge and the application of specific procedures as well as the use of specific terminology on the part of the interpreter. Figure 5.1 (see page 102) lists the multiple functions performed by the interpreter in a variety of contexts.

Maintaining Linguistic Skills

Six linguistic skills are needed to ensure that the interpreter or translator can successfully bridge the communication between two parties who do not share the same language. These skills are applicable to any interpreter or translator working with either a speech-language pathologist or audiologist:

1. Oral or written proficiency with two languages

2. Knowledge of two cultures with an understanding of the significance of nonverbal communication

3. Ability to convey the same meaning in two languages

4. Knowledge of terminology that applies to a designated specialty (speech-language pathology or audiology)

The Interpreter's

Figure 5.1   **Multiple Functions**

Situations

Parent and Family Interviews and Conferences
IEP Team Meetings
Client Observations
Testing and Assessments
Intervention
Due Process Hearings

The Interpreter Bridges Communication between

Speech-language
  pathologists
Audiologists

Families of various
  compositions and
  educational backgrounds

BRIDGING

Various educators
General education teachers
Nurses or other health
  professionals
Hearing officers

Students and patients
  of various ages
  and abilities

5. Familiarity with dialectal differences within a language

6. Ability to adapt to and process various pronunciations and grammatical uses inherent in the speech of individuals with communication disorders

Oral or Written Proficiency with Two Languages

The interpreting process demands the ability to switch languages very quickly and to make rapid adaptations to different personalities, age groups, and levels of formal education. This aspect is even more important in the field of speech-language pathology and audiology given the variety in ages, backgrounds, abilities, and disabilities of both the pediatric and adult populations. Successful interpreting also requires efficient recall of auditory information. If a message is longer than anticipated, the interpreter needs to take notes by writing down keywords and ideas to interpret all that was said.

Competency in the written aspect of the two languages is necessary since the style of writing and, therefore, translation varies from document to document. For example, the style of a letter announcing a field trip is different from the style of an individualized education program (IEP). It is also important for the translator to use correct grammar and spelling in each language to ensure that the meaning is adequately conveyed and that the final product has the necessary professional appearance.

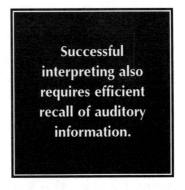

Successful interpreting also requires efficient recall of auditory information.

Today, most commonly spoken languages have a written form. For a review of these different forms, speech-language pathologists and audiologists should consult Campbell (1997). Campbell includes examples for languages such as Bengali, Berber, Burmese, Cambodian, Chinese, Cyrillic, Gujarati, Japanese, and Mongolian.

Knowledge of Two Cultures and Nonverbal Communication

Social and cultural variations need to be considered in the interpreting process. Each situation and context necessitates knowledge of specific vocabulary. In addition, knowledge of dialectal variations for words and pronunciation in general is necessary.

The interpreter must also understand paralinguistic messages such as intonation, use of gestures, and facial expressions of the speakers. As previously discussed, an interpreter is someone who "filters, screens, and amends the message to make it professionally, culturally, and linguistically, appropriate" (Cheng, 1998a, p. 113). The difference between "He performs very well on *these* tasks" and "He performs *very* well on these tasks" needs to be conveyed. The process is further complicated by the fact that the interpreter must be aware of numerous variations in the pronunciation, intonation, and grammar of each language. The interpreter must also interpret the tone or the intent of the message and provide appropriate support of all nonverbal information.

Ability to Convey the Same Meaning in Two Languages

Knowledge of the grammatical and syntactic differences and contrasts between two languages is necessary to ensure accurate translation and interpretation. For example, articles are omitted in certain languages like Chinese, Korean, and Polish. The verb is often placed at the end of a phrase or sentence instead of the middle, as in "I read a book," which is interpreted as "I a book read" in languages like Vietnamese, or when marking the past with a participle as in "Ich habe ein Buch gelesen," "I have a book read" in German. Some languages, like Vietnamese, Japanese, or Chinese, have numerous equivalents for the pronoun *I* depending on a person's status (Cheng, 1991). A more extensive discussion on this topic can be found in Chapter 2 (see "Dialects," page 21).

Knowledge of a Specialty's Terminology

The context and nature of the job necessitates that the interpreter or translator possess specific knowledge of vocabulary and procedures that directly apply to the fields of speech-language pathology and audiology. Terms may be tied to the given context (e.g., a school, a school district, a nursing home, a community center, a hospital, a clinic, or an agency).

When a word does not exist in a language, a definition for a given concept may be necessary. For example, words such as *background, screening, auditory processing,* or *phonemic awareness* do not exist in many languages other than English, so the interpreter or translator must use an alternative word or a group of words to convey a similar meaning in the other language. On the other hand, a word could have two equivalent meanings in another language, and the interpreter or translator must use the correct term for the given situation.

For example, *take* and *cover* (imperative form), which are frequently used in evaluations and intervention procedures, may be conveyed in Spanish as *toma* or *agarra* (take) and *cubre* or *tapa* (cover). The words *agarra/agarre* and *tapa/tape* are used with greater frequency in more informal situations in contrast to the words *toma/tome* and *cubre/cubra*. The word *answer* can be translated as *contestación* or *respuesta*. Each word would be used in a different context. That is, if one were to say, "Answer the following questions," it would be "Contésta/e las siguientes preguntas." However, the word *respuesta* would be used in the context of a reply as in a debate or a conversation where feedback or opinions are needed (e.g., "¿Cuál es tu/su respuesta tocante a la situación en Puerto Rico?" [What is your answer to the current situation in Puerto Rico?]).

In other languages, like French or Polish, there is only one equivalent for the words *take* and *cover*: *prends/prenez* and *wesz/wesz* (take), and *couvrez* and *przykryj* (cover) in the two respective languages. An equivalent word for *answer* (as would be used in a testing situation) exists in each language: *reponds/répondez* (French) and *odpowiedz/odpowiedz* (Polish). Therefore, the interpretation or translation process involves more than providing a word-by-word equivalent, and the interpreter or translator needs to select specific terms to convey a given meaning or intent when switching from one language to the other.

> [T]he interpretation or translation process involves more than providing a word-by-word equivalent.

Specialized or technical terminology occurs in each professional setting. Vocabulary words are connected with a description of procedures such as *individualized educational program*, *least restrictive environment*, *inclusion*, and *due process*. Medical terminology refers to specialized or specific procedures, such as *tracheotomy*, *dysphagia*, *respirator*, *acoustic impedance*, and *auditory brain stem testing*. Some vocabulary is used with greater frequency in a hospital or clinic setting as compared to a school environment.

Therefore, the interpreter or translator needs to be familiar with procedures followed in a given setting where speech-language or audiological services are delivered.

Familiarity with Dialectal Differences

The interpreter or translator should be familiar with dialectal variations and words that have multiple meanings, like the word *grass* that is found in a yard or park. The word has different equivalents in Spanish depending on the specific dialect. Central Americans call it *grama*, Mexicans refer to the word as *pasto*, Spaniards use *cesped*, and Mexican-Americans call it *zacate*. A clinician once reported that a Nicaraguan child was unable to provide the correct response to a verbal analogy because the child had not understood the word *zacate*. Other considerations include understanding differences in grammatical and syntactic constructions between two languages and being sensitive to variation in speech patterns. The latter is especially important in the fields of speech-language pathology and audiology because a great majority of individuals are seen for a communication disorder that may be reflected in unusual speech and language patterns.

Ability to Adapt to the Speech and Language of People with Communication Disorders

Careful interpretation is particularly important during an assessment. In this situation, the individual's responses must be interpreted verbatim, without editorializing. For example, if a child says *gande* instead of *grande* (big), and *ápiz* instead of *lápiz* (pencil), the interpreter must communicate the word in the same way it was pronounced. Accurate interpretation is also necessary in recording longer utterances such as "El cado se paró frente a tienda" (the caw stopped front of store), instead of the correct form "El carro se paró en frente de la tienda" (the car stopped in front of the store). The interpreter must have an understanding of the speech-language pathologist's need to determine whether an error such as *cado/carro* is phonologically or lexically based.

Following a Code of Ethics

A code of ethics for interpreters who work with communication disorders professionals has not been developed, but codes exist for others, including interpreters working in the United Nations, with the deaf, in the courts, and in the medical professions. The Overview of Role and Practice Issues (Diversity Rx, 1997) identified role and practice issues related to interpreting in the medical and allied-health fields. The Registry of Interpreters for the Deaf (2001) established ethical standards for interpreters of American Sign Language and English in the United States. The Australian Institute of Interpreters and Translators (AUSIT, 2000) is the professional organization that identified ethical standards for those practicing in Australia.

ASHA (1998) indicated that assistants used as interpreters and translators should be adequately trained and meet minimum competencies in order to provide the highest quality of service to multicultural populations. The code of ethics proposed in the sidebar on page 110 includes key considerations for the interpreter or translator working with communication disorders professionals.

Maintaining Neutrality and Confidentiality

The interpreter serves as a bridge between two or more parties to interpret everything that is being said, including offensive and negative remarks, to make the communication process successful. Also, the interpreter must understand the particular characteristics of a given culture or group, without making assumptions based on stereotypes. The interpreter can provide the speech-language pathologist or audiologist with helpful insights on various topics such as child-rearing practices, self-help and knowledge-based expectations for children of various ages, and family dynamics. For example, it is not unusual in some Mexican families for young children to be dressed and bathed by their parents well into their fourth or fifth year of life, so children do not develop early independence in these self-help skills. They may also converse more with siblings than with parents. In some cultures, a disability may be equated to being sick. A more specific example includes Fadiman's (1997) comments in interpreting how a Hmong family might understand a physician's questions about their daughter's early seizures:

> 1-*What do you call the problem?*
> *Quag dag peg.* That means the spirit catches you
> and you fall down.

> 2-*What do you think caused the problem?*—
> Soul loss.

> 3-*Why do you think it started when it did?*
> Lia's sister Yer slammed the door and Lia's soul
> was frightened out of her body. (p. 260)

Code of Ethics for Interpreters Working in Speech-Language Pathology and Audiology

1. Be certified through formal training.

2. Accept work or assignments only where linguistically and culturally competent.

3. Be adequately prepared for a given assignment.

4. Interpret the message, the material, or the interaction accurately.

5. Keep the information conveyed confidential.

6. Ask for clarification from the speech-language or audiologist, the client, the parent, the family member, or any other participant if uncertain about the meaning of a message, document, or interaction.

7. Decline a job where there might be a conflict of interest.

8. Refrain from providing independent advice or information without consultation or guidance from the communication disorders professional.

9. Be punctual in responding to various assignments or attending meetings.

10. Show respect for all parties involved.

11. Continue professional development in the field of interpretation and in aspects of speech-language pathology and audiology.

For more information on child-rearing practices and parental expectations, speech-language pathologists and audiologists are referred to sources such as Cheng (1991), Langdon (1992a), and van Kleeck (1994).

The interpreter needs to remain neutral about behaviors or statements that reflect the client's culture or background. Knowledge and understanding of similarities and differences between two cultures enables the interpreter to provide more accurate interpretations of what

> **The interpreter needs to remain neutral about behaviors or statements that reflect the client's culture or background.**

is being said. The interpreter can assist the communication disorders professional by sharing all relevant cultural information in a nonjudgemental way. The interpreter must also respect the confidentiality that is inherent in the process. For example, the interpreter should not discuss a case with other members of the community or other professionals outside the professional setting.

Interpreting Faithfully

When a Chinese speaker says "ni fa fu le," which literally means "you have gained weight," the interpreter should use the expression "you look healthy" instead of providing a word-by-word interpretation, which would not convey the correct intent of the utterance (Cheng, 1998a, p. 115). This type of interpretation demonstrates that the interpreter understands the cultural implications of the message.

Because the underlying meaning must be conveyed, interpreting idioms is particularly difficult. For example, it is not accurate to literally interpret an idiom such as "con toda confianza" (with all confidence); instead, the interpreter should use "feel free." Likewise, they may not word-by-word interpret the Spanish idiom "cayó redondo al suelo" (she fell round on the floor), but instead, "she fell flat on the floor." In this case, *redondo* (round) needs to be interpreted as *flat*. Thus, interpreting specific terminology and idioms requires in-depth knowledge of two linguistic systems and two cultures. When an accurate or equivalent rendering of an idiom cannot be provided, an explanation of the idiom in the alternate language may be necessary.

Interpreters must be careful to present standardized and non-standardized assessment tasks according to accepted procedures. The interpreter should avoid the use of unnecessary gestures, intonation, or any cues that would guide a client toward a given response during the testing process. However, the use of cues, repetition, and scaffolding may be important in the intervention process when used with the knowledge and direction of the communication disorders professional.

Participating in Ongoing Learning and Remaining Flexible

The interpreter should respond positively to constructive criticisms and suggestions to foster increased job effectiveness. Each interpreter must remain current about new procedures specified by a given school, medical agency, or collaborating specialist. For example, different procedures are used by speech-language pathologists in school, clinic, hospital, or long-term-care settings. Specific steps and strategies are followed in assessing the hearing status of patients of different ages. The interpreter should be responsive to the directions of the audiologist in making adjustments for different ages.

State-certified deaf interpreters, court interpreters, and medical interpreters must earn a given number of continuing education units to retain their certification. Interpreters working with speech-language pathologists and audiologists should remain current as well. In any case, interpreters should avoid performing tasks that may be too difficult, or for which insufficient training and experience have been provided. As explained in the previous sections, the interpreter must balance many roles. Table 5.1 summarizes these roles.

Table 5.1   **Summary of an Interpreter's Roles**

Do	Don't
Act ethically	Assume you should help whenever called
Remain neutral	Take over the role of the communication disorders professional
Respect confidentiality	Discuss a case outside the given setting
Interpret faithfully	Provide cues when not called for
Become a lifelong learner	Accept jobs that are too difficult

THREE IMPORTANT STEPS: BRIEFING, INTERACTION, AND DEBRIEFING (BID)

The success of the interpreting process for conferences, interviews with families or clients, assessments, or intervention is enhanced when it includes the three steps of briefing, interaction, and debriefing (BID). Videos by Cheng, Langdon, and Davies (1991) and Langdon (in press) illustrate these steps for conferences and assessments respectively.

The three-step process provides the speech-language pathologist or audiologist with adequate time to collaborate with the interpreter. Preparation and evaluation of the conference, assessment, or intervention session are essential elements.

> The...process provides the speech-language pathologist or audiologist with adequate time to collaborate with the interpreter.

Briefing is the initial step. The speech-language pathologist or audiologist takes time with the interpreter to formulate the agenda for a given conference, assessment session, or intervention session. During this time, decisions about simultaneous or consecutive interpreting are made (see "Methods of Interpreting and Translating," page 15). The communication disorders professional should describe the purpose and desired outcomes of the session, and the interpreter should provide input on methods that will facilitate the process.

Interaction constitutes the next step and includes the actual time that the speech-language pathologist or audiologist and the interpreter work together in a conference, assessment session, or intervention session. The speech-language pathologist or audiologist should address the parent or client directly, rather than addressing the interpreter. The interpreter should transmit what is said by all parties as accurately as possible. The interpreter and the speech-language pathologist or audiologist should work collaboratively and maintain a united team.

During the *debriefing* period, the interpreter and the speech-language pathologist or audiologist review the outcomes of the conference, assessment session, or intervention session. The team reviews the dynamics of the conference or the client's responses to specific materials. Follow-up plans are also outlined during this period.

BID During Interviews and Conferences

Figure 5.2 (see page 116) is a checklist of areas to consider when following the BID steps in collaboration with an interpreter during interviews and conferences. Areas to consider are listed under each one of the three steps of briefing, interaction, and debriefing. This form may be duplicated.

The interpreter should interpret all statements using the first person. For example, if a parent says "I have been concerned about my child," the interpreter presents the statement as is, without saying "Mrs. X says that..."

Collaboration with an Interpreter in

Figure 5.2 **Interviews or Conferences: A Checklist**

Briefing		
Format of the interview or conference is explained	Y	N
Purpose of the interview or conference is explained	Y	N
Critical pieces of information are reviewed	Y	N
Critical questions are reviewed (where applicable)	Y	N
Type of interpreting (consecutive or simultaneous) is discussed	Y	N
Comments: _____		
_____		
Interaction		
Seating arrangement is appropriate	Y	N
Communication disorders professional introduces participants	Y	N
Communication disorders professional defines roles	Y	N
Communication disorders professional states the purpose of the conference	Y	N
Interpreter interprets using "I" instead of "Mr. X says"	Y	N
Interpreter transmits all that the parent says	Y	N
Team maintains eye contact with the parent (if culturally appropriate)	Y	N
Team's language is understandable to the parent	Y	N

Figure 5.2—*Continued*

Team appears ultimately responsible for the conference procedure, information sharing, and intent	Y	N
Team presents itself as a unit	Y	N
Environment is comfortable	Y	N
Attention is paid to nonverbal cues	Y	N
Interpreter interprets clearly and precisely	Y	N
Interpreter asks for clarification when necessary	Y	N

Comments:_____

_____

Debriefing

Was the interview or conference productive?	Y	N

Areas that went well: _____

_____

Areas to emphasize in the future:_____

_____

Comments:_____

_____

Communication disorders professionals should direct all comments to the parent, student, or client, not to the interpreter. This allows participants to feel that all messages are addressed directly to them. However, this strategy can be difficult to implement because either party may feel uncomfortable communicating to one another through another person, the interpreter.

In some instances, family members may understand more English than they are willing to admit. Family members may be asked if they wish to use the interpreter's services. While they may understand most English, they may want to make sure they understand all the details, and may feel more comfortable speaking in the language in which they are most fluent.

Family members and patients may not understand the laws and regulations that guarantee their rights. Procedures for informing them and gaining their written consent may be unfamiliar or unsettling. Requesting that these individuals summarize the main points is a helpful technique to ascertain that they indeed understand the essence of their rights. The authors recommend that parents check a box on the IEP indicating that they understand their rights as parents of a student with special needs.

Family members and clients must understand the results of assessments, recommendations, and intervention plans. Family members often fail to question what the school or the health professional is saying. This attitude is common in individuals who were raised in countries where advice of professionals is accepted unconditionally. Families and clients need to have time and opportunity to assimilate the process. Additional time may be needed for families to agree to an assessment or intervention and this should be respected. Naturally, there might be situations where an agreement from the family is needed immediately (e.g., when requesting permission to perform an endoscopy). The communication disorders professional needs to communicate very clearly the reason for urgency in making such a decision.

It is not unusual for a family to bring an advocate who is bilingual to a meeting. Establishing a positive attitude from the start is key to a successful outcome. For example, the process can be facilitated if the speech-language pathologist or audiologist begins the meeting by stating the role of each member and by indicating that comments from the bilingual advocate are welcome. The interpreter will continue to interpret all comments from all participants. The members of the conference team should convey that they are working as a unit. Ultimately, all parties involved need to understand that the conference is carried out to benefit the client and that the communication disorders professional is the person who is legally responsible for the outcome of the conference.

Keep in mind that in some cultures, making direct eye contact is avoided as a sign of respect. The professional should be sensitive to the family's background and culture and behave accordingly (Harry, 1992; Pang and Cheng, 1998).

Seating arrangements are also important. The interpreter should sit next to the parent, family member, or client. One person at a time should speak. Side conversations between members of a given team who are participating in the interview or conference should be avoided. The speech-language pathologist or audiologist and the interpreter should be sensitive to the reactions of the client and the family member, and they need to be certain that messages are clearly conveyed. The interpreter should transmit everything that is said, including every one of the participant's responses, comments, questions, requests for clarification, or repetitions.

When the interview or conference is completed, the communication disorders professional and the interpreter should take time to evaluate what went well and how the process might be improved in the future. Follow-up plans should be developed.

In summary, the interpreter and the communication disorders professional should ensure that the environment supports the parent or family in feeling like a part of the process. Using the first person while interpreting what each party says, maintaining eye contact with all parties to the extent that it is culturally appropriate, addressing each party and not the interpreter, arranging seating properly, and avoiding side conversations will support the process.

BID during Assessment and Intervention

Figure 5.3 lists areas to be addressed in making assessment and intervention successful. This form may be duplicated. To facilitate the process, the interpreter should have met the client prior to an assessment. This may not be possible in some settings, because the client may be seen during an emergency or may be unavailable at other times. In any event, the interpreter should be briefed as much as possible about pertinent aspects of a client's background and should be familiar with the assessment procedures and tests.

Regardless of preparation, the interpreter should not test an individual without the presence of the speech-language pathologist or audiologist. Even though the interpreter may be the major person interacting during the assessment process, it

Collaboration with an Interpreter in
Figure 5.3 **Assessment or Intervention: A Checklist**

Briefing		
Purpose of the assessment or intervention is explained	Y	N
Procedures to be followed are reviewed	Y	N
Use of gestures, voice patterns, and other body language that might cue the client are discussed	Y	N
The interpreter is reminded to write down all relevant information and keep notes	Y	N
The communication disorders professional has test protocols to follow during the assessment	Y	N
There is evidence that the interpreter has interacted with the client prior to the session (variable)	Y	N
There is evidence that the communication disorders professional has interacted with the client prior to the session	Y	N

Comments:_____

_____

Interaction		
Communication disorders professional is present	Y	N
Interpreter asks questions immediately as needed	Y	N
Communication disorders professional takes notes	Y	N

Note Relevant Client Behaviors

Displays general behavior problems such as perseveration, short attention span, distractibility	Y	N
Needs repetition and cuing	Y	N
Uses more gestures than words to express ideas	Y	N

Continued on next page

Figure 5.3—*Continued*

Has difficulty with language skills such as pauses, hesitations,
    response delays, reauditorization, short answers   Y   N

Benefits from various strategies such as repetition,
    modeling, breaking down information   Y   N

Comments on other behaviors observed:_____

_____

Note Relevant Interpreter Behaviors

Uses appropriate nonverbal communication   Y   N

Gives clear instructions   Y   N

Provides adequate reinforcement   Y   N

Cues or prompts the client where appropriate   Y   N

Takes notes   Y   N

Asks for information from the communication
    disorders professional when needed   Y   N

Comments:_____

_____

Debriefing

Client's responses are reviewed   Y   N

Interpreter relates what the client should or should not
    have said in response to specific questions   Y   N

Any difficulties in the process are reviewed   Y   N

Language sample is documented, annotated,
    and reviewed   Y   N

Comments:_____

_____

Materials used for assessment or intervention: _____

_____

is vital that the speech-language pathologist or audiologist be present to observe the interaction, to direct the interpreter, and to be available to clarify directions or interpretations of a test item. The interpreter and the speech-language pathologist or audiologist can also confer on what actions to take in case the client does not cooperate or experiences more or less difficulty in responding to specific tasks than had been anticipated.

Depending on the particular test or test items, the situation, and the interpreter's level of training and experience, the interpreter may proceed by asking the client to respond to the items without needing the speech-language pathologist or audiologist to administer the given item(s) using English first. The process is facilitated if the speech-language pathologist refers back to the specific test protocols in the client's first language. The procedures to follow when tests in a given language are not available are discussed in Chapter 4. These suggestions also apply to the intervention process. In the latter case, the presence of the speech-language pathologist enables the interpreter to modify or shift strategies during intervention in case the client responds differently than anticipated.

The speech-language pathologist or audiologist and the interpreter must agree on the procedure they will follow ahead of time. The particular tests with specific beginning-item administration and order of presentation should be discussed in testing speech, language, and communication skills. When assessing the client's hearing acuity, for example, it is important that the client understands that he or she needs to respond even when tones are very faint. At times, assessing the client while using masking becomes very difficult because the patient does not understand the procedure of the test. When no interpreter is available, some experienced audiologists demonstrate to the patient what he or she needs to do using gestures and the portable audiometer prior to proceeding to the testing booth (J. Lang and J. McCullough, personal communication, April 12, 2000). Understanding directions and feeling at ease are very important in getting an accurate measure of the client's hearing acuity. Thus, adequate preparation of the interpreter during the briefing is important to ensure the success of the process.

The interpreter should not leave immediately after the conclusion of a session. Following the assessment, the team of interpreter and speech-language pathologist or audiologist should review the different points that were discussed, evaluate the results, and plan the

> [A]dequate preparation of the interpreter during the briefing is important to ensure the success of the process.

necessary follow-up. They should be certain that the family's questions and legal rights were addressed adequately. Sufficient time should be set aside to review the client's assessment results. The language sample should be transcribed and then translated into English with notations about the client's specific strengths and challenges in language comprehension and expression. Both team members should share and discuss their observations.

An outline of areas to improve at subsequent sessions should be delineated. Although the interpreter's role is important in every step of the process, all parties should remember that the speech-language pathologist or audiologist is the professional who is ultimately responsible for the outcome of the assessment as well as for its follow-up for speech, language, hearing, and communication services. The written report should document that the assessment took place in collaboration with the interpreter. The role of each team member should be described. This includes documentation of the materials used, the procedures followed in recording results, and a statement about the validity of the results obtained. A sample report is included in Appendix D.

If the collaboration of an interpreter is necessary during intervention, a continuous dialogue should take place between the interpreter and the speech-language pathologist. The interpreter, under the direction of the speech-language pathologist, can assist the client in gaining specific language and communication skills in the primary language. Subsequently, the speech-language pathologist can introduce the same concepts in English once it is determined that the client is able to comprehend sufficient English to respond to intervention in that language. The interpreter, under the direction of the speech-language pathologist, will be asked to provide the client's family with specific suggestions for activities to follow up with at home. To ensure that parents or families understand their role in helping the client at home, the speech-language pathologist will need to ask them to explain it using their own words. The interpreter will in turn need to interpret what the family members or parents said to ensure that the messages were clearly understood. Similarly, the interpreter's role is very important during counseling regarding the use and care of particular equipment and hearing aids for the client who is hearing impaired or deaf.

Enhancing Professional Development Programs and the Future of Interpreters

6

Confusion and inconsistency in the minds of both the trainees and trainers in their understanding of the parameters of the role of the cultural interpreter [was a key issue in a Training Symposium in Ontario in 1992].

—M. Giovannini

Chapter Goals

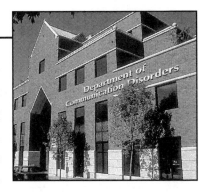

- Review the areas of difficulty that may prevent interpreters from working in specialized fields, including inconsistencies in professional development programs, lack of proficiency in two languages, low pay, and inconsistent hours

- Outline a professional development program designed specifically for interpreters working with speech-language pathologists and audiologists

- Provide checklists, which may be duplicated, for speech-language pathologists, audiologists, interpreters, and consumers to use when evaluating their collaboration

- Suggest some activities that may help illuminate the future of interpreters in speech-language pathology and audiology

DISCUSSION ITEMS

1. What are two things that could be done to improve the areas of difficulty that may prevent interpreters from working in specialized fields?

2. What criteria would you use for selecting participants in a training program for interpreters in communication disorders?

3. Should communication disorders professionals attend a training program along with interpreters? How much time should each member of the collaborative team devote to an initial training program?

4. Role-play an evaluation meeting between an interpreter and a speech-language pathologist or audiologist using Figure 6.1 (page 147) as a guide.

5. Which of the suggested research areas on pages 151 and 154–156 would be most useful in your current or future work setting? Briefly describe how you could carry out or contribute to this research and how it would benefit your practice or the field.

AREAS OF DIFFICULTY FOR INTERPRETERS

Inconsistencies in Professional Development Programs

The field of interpreting in allied health, education, or social service has not received the same recognition as international interpreting, court interpreting, or interpreting for the deaf. The need for interpreter services has not been fully acknowledged. This lack of recognition is related to the lack of certification of graduates of professional development programs.

The success of interpreting programs for specialized fields has been variable due to inconsistency in their scope or duration (Roberts, 1997). University programs often have goals that are focused on the courts or the international arena, which are different than goals for community-based interpreters (Carr, 1997). Many university programs focus on international interpreting, which is different from interpreting in contexts such as medical, clinical, or allied-health professions (Pochhacker, 1997). Training for the latter purposes has consisted of continuing education programs in large universities. These programs have not been part of a rigorous, established program and have lacked professional status (Gehrke, 1993). Training has most often been offered by service providers (e.g., individual hospitals or school districts), resulting in inconsistencies regarding the goals of the program and follow-up training. Flores, Martin, and Champlin (1996) surveyed audiologists in the five states with the largest Hispanic populations (New Mexico,

129

California, Texas, Arizona, and Colorado). Only 18% reported they could provide services in Spanish, and 80% provided services with some help. Of those needing help, 50% asked a family member to interpret, and 30% relied on a co-worker to interpret. This example illustrates the unavailability of interpreters and the lack of consistency in training and preparation of interpreters.

> **Graduates of existing programs are often not given the professional status they deserve.**

The lack of rigorous professional development programs for interpreters working in allied-health professions or community-based organizations has negatively affected efforts to conduct research on the effectiveness of interpreters (Roberts, 1997). Graduates of existing programs are often not given the professional status they deserve. In addition, the limited success of interpreter programs is attributed to the lack of education and involvement of the professionals who use interpreter services (Corsellis, 1997; Nicholson and Martinsen, 1997; Roberts, 1997). In a program designed for speech-language pathology assistants, Manuel-Dupont and Yoakum (1997) concluded that both communication disorders professionals and interpreters need to work together to ensure the success of the process.

Professional development programs need to be certified or accredited so that their graduates may be recognized. These programs should advocate for official recognition of the interpreting profession by working with state agencies that license or certify personnel in school and health-care settings.

Lack of Proficiency in Two Languages

The process of interpreting has often been of inferior quality because of interpreters' inadequate linguistic skills in one or both languages. Often, personnel seeking this type of job are immigrants themselves, and they may not have sufficient skills in English or their native language to fulfill their duties adequately (Benmaman, 1997). Manuel-Dupont and Yoakum (1997) reported that 8 of the 22 candidates for their interpreter education program were unable to complete the program due lack of proficiency in either their native language or English. Most of the programs have been available only in English because training in other languages is often very expensive (Roberts, 1997). It is clear that people wishing to become interpreters need to be highly proficient in both languages and be bicultural in order to succeed in the profession (Benmaman, 1997; Mikkelson and Mintz, 1997).

Low Pay and Inconsistent Hours

Another reason for fewer numbers of trained interpreters in the allied-health professions is a low salary schedule given the responsibilities and skills needed to perform their duties adequately. Organizations that need the services of interpreters and society at large must understand that services provided by interpreters cannot be carried out on low salaries or on a volunteer basis (Fortier, 1997). Furthermore, the overall low number of full-time positions and the variable or unpredictable hours of employment (services needed in emergency cases in any given agency) make the profession unattractive to skilled workers.

Collaborating with an interpreter requires additional time and this should be factored into the duties of the speech-language pathologist or audiologist. Administrators may need to be convinced about this important issue in calculating budgets since additional time for the process is often not factored into costs. With cutbacks in health-care funding, the services of interpreters have been cut drastically compared to just a few years ago, as reported by an audiologist who has been working in a county hospital (J. Lang, personal communication, April 12, 2000).

DESIGNING A PROFESSIONAL DEVELOPMENT PROGRAM

There are currently few professional development programs available for interpreters and communication disorders professionals to learn their collaborative roles. The hypothetical program proposed here could vary depending on the professional and linguistic background of the individuals who participate. This program could be implemented at a university or technical college. Speech-language pathologists, audiologists, interpreters, and translators could attend such a program. Specific guidelines regarding recruitment and training of interpreters and speech-language pathologists and audiologists are described in this section. .

Set a criteria for the program candidates—Candidates should be proficient in the two languages in which they perform their duties, and they should understand characteristics and variations of the two cultures. People already in training or licensed as speech-language pathology assistants and nurses aides may be especially interested in this program.

Establish minimum criteria for linguistic proficiency in both the oral and written areas of two languages—Mikkelson and Mintz (1997) report that certain states, such as Washington and New Jersey, have implemented rigorous language exams for court interpreters. In California, there are exams only for Spanish and English court and medical interpreters. Examinations consist of multiple-choice questions that are related to general vocabulary and word usage, grammar, reading comprehension, and translations of medical and other related vocabulary from English to Spanish and vice versa. An oral language proficiency examination is also performed. The examination is tape-recorded and appraised by two examiners. Testing includes consecutive and simultaneous interpreting in addition to sight translation. The candidate's performance is assessed in both interpreting skills and in mastery of language skills. The examination is graded pass or fail (California State Personnel Board, 1998–2000).

Set criteria for the program—Criteria have already been established in court interpreting, medical interpreting, and deaf interpreting, but only in a few states. For example, inconsistencies in the selection process and training of potential medical interpreters continue to exist (Diversity Rx, 1997). Consolidation of criteria is therefore necessary. For example, programs should include opportunities to develop short-term memory skills, note-taking skills, consecutive interpreting with scripts, knowledge of most commonly used phrases and typical sentences, knowledge of terminology specific to the profession, and use of technology in translation (e.g., machine translation and online dictionaries).

An exit examination should be used to validate the proficiency of the candidate (Benmaman, 1997). Michael and Cocchini (1997) describe a program that has been offered to bilingual students at Hunter College in New York. The training provided students with activities to enhance their interpreting and translating skills following the suggestions given by Benmaman. The training included a review of a code of ethics, role-play exercises using videotapes, journal writing to promote reflections, and in-class discussions. The purpose of the program was not to train students to become professional medical interpreters, but for the students to gain a better understanding of interpreting and translating and to strengthen the students' bilingual skills. The existing literature has focused on educating interpreters and translators, but not those who collaborate with them.

Some literature describing the requirements for interpreters working with speech-language pathologists and audiologists and educational personnel has been available for quite some time (Fradd, 1993; Langdon, Siegel, Halog, and Sánchez-Boyce, 1994; Toliver-Weddington and Meyerson, 1983). There has been scant information, though, describing the actual implementation of a program for such professionals, with the exception of Matsuda and O'Connor (1993) and Manuel-Dupont and Yoakum (1997). See the sidebar for more information on these programs.

Two Reported Professional Development Programs

Matsuda and O'Connor
Department of Communicative Disorders,
California State University, Los Angeles, CA

Twelve hours of class included a discussion of basics in interpreting, applications to assessment and intervention, and general knowledge of second language development. To qualify for the program, the interpreter passed a language examination that included a written translation and a sight translation of a certain passage in both English and the native language. An oral interview was required for English only.

Manuel-Dupont and Yoakum
Utah State University and Granite School District
Salt Lake City, Utah

Phase 1 included 12 Saturday sessions over a three-month period. The 20 participants took courses that included normal speech and language acquisition; disorders of speech, language, and hearing; behavior management; materials for intervention; and professional ethics. Participants had little opportunity to implement the knowledge they acquired in the classroom, and many dropped out of the program.

Phase 2 dropped some of the academic requirements to enable the participants to gain more practical experience. This three-weekend program of 21 hours included a brief review of the material covered in Phase I and ample time for practice in translation to make participants more aware of their two languages.

Continued on next page

Two Reported Professional Development Programs—*Continued*

In Phase 3, new candidates were recruited because of some difficulties in maintaining interest and commitment from the original participants. The program focused more on practicing the candidate's current language abilities, an aspect that had not been considered before. The program ran for 8 Saturdays, with each session lasting 4–6 hours, and focused on the translation and interpreting process; child development; case history data gathering techniques; problems associated with using standardized language tests in assessing culturally/linguistically diverse (CLD) populations; contrasts in normal language development across cultures; techniques in informal assessment, including narratives; and dynamic assessment techniques.

Minimum Qualifications for Program Participants

Content Knowledge

Candidates desiring to become interpreters in communication disorders professions should have a solid foundation in speech and language development, speech-language and hearing disorders, clinical management, and assistive technology.

One ideal pool of candidates would be those who are bilingual and are pursuing a career as speech-language pathology assistants. Another pool could be nurses aides who want to specialize in assisting audiologists and otolaryngologists. At this time, for example, three programs have been officially recognized by the Medical Board of Examiners in Speech-Pathology and Audiology in California as institutions that train speech-language pathology assistants: Evergreen College in San José, California and Pasadena Community College and Cerritos College in the Los Angeles area. The first two programs were initiated in the fall of 1999, while the third one began in the fall of 2000. Students in the Evergreen College program take a number of courses that are similar to, but in lesser depth, those required for a bachelor's degree in speech-language pathology in most ASHA accredited speech-language pathology programs in California.

Proficiency in Two Languages

The candidate seeking interpreter credentials must fulfill a minimum bilingual language requirement, as verified through a formal examination. An example examination may proceed in the following manner. Initially, each candidate must pass an oral and written examination in both English and their non-English language (NEL) to assess their linguistic skills. Special language teachers may have to be hired to assess the candidate's linguistic skills. An examination similar to the scale proposed by the Foreign Service Institute, which is based on a scale of 1 to 5 (with 3 being the minimum standard accepted to perform a given professional task), may be used for the oral portion of the examination (Skehan, 1988). Written language skills may be assessed by asking the candidate to write a short essay on a given topic related to education (e.g., writing a letter to a parent announcing a meeting or summarizing the content of an IEP in both English and the NEL). The essay could be scored holistically and through various rubrics to evaluate ability to convey meaning, sentence formulation, punctuation, and spelling. In addition, each candidate may be asked to translate a portion of a report on a client from English to the NEL and to translate a letter written by a parent or family member describing their child's or relative's communication difficulty. Obtaining results from these assessments assists the program leaders in identifying specific areas to emphasize in the translating portion of the program.

Professional Development Program Description

General Components

To ensure the success of the professional development program, both the interpreters and the communication disorders professionals working with them are required to attend. This enables both parties to receive the same basic information and to work collaboratively on various assignments. Pairing the interpreter with a speech-language pathologist or audiologist strengthens the quality of the program by ensuring that the interpreter becomes familiar with the policies of a given school, agency, clinic, or hospital. The interpreter becomes familiar with procedures that are followed from the time a student is referred to the time the IEP team meeting is conducted, from the time a patient is admitted for a given procedure to the time of discharge, or from the time a client seeks an audiological exam through aural rehabilitation, if needed.

Interpreters receive certification following completion of course requirements and a final examination. Speech-language pathologists and audiologists receive continuing education units (CEUs) for ASHA, their state license, or both and may receive graduate credit for advancement on their agency's salary schedule. The following basic areas are addressed:

1. Roles and responsibilities of the interpreter and the speech-language pathologist or audiologist, including a code of ethics

2. Specific procedures inherent to the particular profession and policies followed in the given setting, such as school, clinic, or hospital

3. The process of interpretation and translation

4. Locations of necessary materials and references

5. Simulations using various scenarios (e.g., conferences, gathering background information, assessments, and intervention) where speech-language pathologists, audiologists, and interpreters practice using their skills together

> **Interpreters receive certification following completion of course requirements and a final examination.**

Sessions extend over a three- to five-month period. This enables the participants to practice the information presented at each session and promotes discussions and reflections at subsequent sessions about the various issues that emerge in the process of interpreting and translating.

Implementation issues are discussed as part of the training. The interpreter practices administering a given assessment procedure before serving as the interpreter. The speech-language pathologist or audiologist helps the interpreter obtain various materials, such as dictionaries and access to the Internet, to search specific references and resources in any given language. One useful resource is the National Clearinghouse of Bilingual Education (www.ncbe.gwu.edu/links/langcult/linguistics.html), which includes links to Spanish, Vietnamese, Hmong, Korean, Native American, Chinese, and Tagalog languages. Numerous resources are available under each language. Links to educational resources, organizations, and web indexes of resources are provided for each language.

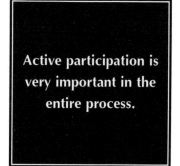

Active participation is very important in the entire process.

A Proposed Syllabus

The ideal professional development program for preparing interpreters that is proposed by the authors and outlined in the following sections takes place over a five-month period with meetings occurring once a month for 9 hours each (over a two-day period) for a total of 45 hours of classroom time. Three hours of class time are delivered on Friday evening and six hours on Saturday. An additional 15 hours is factored in for various outside assignments, so the total training takes 60 hours. Specific topics are covered in each session. Active participation is very important in the entire process. Each team (speech-language pathologist and interpreter or audiologist and interpreter) participates and works together in completing and presenting assignments.

Classes are taught by interpreters who have worked in communication disorders fields for at least two years and speech-language pathologists and audiologists who have collaborated with them. Curriculum and goals are shared by all instructors. This book; the accompanying manual by Langdon (2002); and the videotapes by Cheng, Langdon, and Davies (1991) and Langdon (in press) are used as materials for the program. Participants must be present at all sessions and must complete all assignments in a timely and complete fashion. A point system is used to appraise the quality of the assignments, and participants must receive a certain number of points to graduate.

Receiving a certification equivalent to that awarded to conference interpreters, interpreters for the deaf, court interpreters, and medical interpreters enables interpreters working with speech-language pathologists, audiologists, and other education or health-care personnel to gain the professional status they deserve.

First Month: The Process of Interpreting and Translating

Topics

1. Definitions of interpretation and translation

2. Attributes, roles, and responsibilities of an interpreter, including a code of ethics

3. Roles and responsibilities of a speech-language pathologist and audiologist

4. The role of an interpreter in interviews and conferences

5. Videotape critique (Cheng, Langdon, and Davies, 1991)

6. Simulations and role-plays

7. Practice of short-term memory skills, note-taking skills, and consecutive interpreting with scripts

8. Terminology in the professions of speech-language pathology and audiology

9. Tools and resources, including machine translation and online reference sources

Assignment

The assignment consists of three steps (to be completed by each team of speech-language pathologist and interpreter or audiologist and interpreter):

1. Videotape a speech-language pathologist or audiologist working with an interpreter during one of the following situations: a parent conference about an English language learning (ELL) student who may be referred for a speech-language assessment or an audiological examination, a culturally/linguistically diverse (CLD) client who is seen for an audiological examination, or a client's relative who is interviewed because the client has sustained an injury affecting his or her ability to communicate effectively. (Teams must obtain the necessary permission to tape.)

2. Edit the videotape to show important segments, and be prepared to make a 15-minute oral presentation to the class the following month.

3. Submit a written report of no more than four pages discussing the case, describing the procedures followed, and indicating what was accomplished in the process. Make recommendations about what might be done next time to improve the outcome of the interaction.

Second Month: Collaboration with an Interpreter in Assessing CLD Clients

Topics

1. Discussion of the videotaped demonstrations brought by class participants

2. Assessment of CLD populations from various perspectives, including information that needs to be collected prior to or during the assessment

3. Methods of assessment in speech, language, and hearing

4. Advantages and disadvantages of standardized tests

5. Critique of tests available in various languages

6. Issues surrounding translating tests into other languages

7. Review of assessment procedures in audiology

Note: Teams may need to be separated into a speech-language pathology group and an audiology group to focus on available tests in their respective disciplines.

Assignment

The assignment consists of presenting a case where a test was available in the primary language. Teams give a 15-minute oral presentation to describe the case and the methods used in assessing the client's speech, language, communication, or hearing.

Third Month: Assessment of CLD Clients

Topics

1. Plans for assessment of clients when tests are not available in the target language

2. Role of dynamic assessment

3. Administration and analysis of a language sample

4. Successful methods in assessing hearing and auditory processing

5. Video critique (Langdon, in press)

6. Discussion of participants' cases from the second month assignment, comparing and contrasting procedures used and discussing what could have been done differently

Note: As in the previous month, speech-language pathologists and audiologists may need to be separated to focus on procedures specific to their respective disciplines.

Assignment

Teams videotape and report on a case study where the assessment techniques shared in class are implemented. In this case, in contrast to the second assignment, emphasis is on describing situations where there are no available tests in a given language. (Teams must obtain the necessary permission to tape.)

Fourth Month: Other Roles Fulfilled by Interpreters in Communication Disorders Professions

Topics

1. Discussion of participants' cases from the third-month assignment

2. Challenges of translation

3. Speech-language intervention with CLD clients

4. Aural rehabilitation with CLD clients

5. Prescription and testing of a hearing aid

6. Case studies

Assignment

Teams report on a case where interpreters assisted in the delivery of services and answer the following questions:

- How did other team members interface with the interpreter? What were each team member's responsibilities?

- What process was used in any of the following situations: an IEP; a conference with a client or relative regarding the client's speech, language, or hearing status; or an intervention session?

Teams then complete a one- or two-page summary of the interaction written in English and a translation of the summary in the primary language of the client.

Fifth Month: Outcome of the Program

Topics

1. Discussion of previous month's assignments

2. Evaluation of the each team member's performance

3. Evaluation of team skills

4. Plan for working with administrators to ensure that interpreters are adequately compensated

5. Written reflections about training (each team will respond to a set of questions to evaluate what they learned and how they will continue to implement what they learned)

6. Course evaluation

On-the-Job Evaluation

It is important that speech-language pathologists and audiologists have objective ways to measure an interpreter's performance and provide meaningful feedback. The checklist in Figure 6.1 may be used to indicate the interpreter's performance. Keeping an ongoing record of the interpreter's performance enables the speech-language pathologist or audiologist and the interpreter to focus on specific areas to ensure that the process of interpreting and translating is adequately performed.

In addition, a special evaluation form may be used for parents, relatives, and others who have used the services of the interpreter. Figure 6.2 (see pages 149–150) is adapted from suggestions by

Evaluation of
Figure 6.1   **the Interpreter's Skills**

Key: (1) Always   (2) Often   (3) Sometimes   (4) Rarely   (5) Never

GENERAL BEHAVIORS

1. Does the interpreter ask questions to find out
   what is planned for a given meeting?   1   2   3   4   5

2. Does the interpreter seek clarification
   when something is ambiguous?   1   2   3   4   5

3. Does the interpreter listen carefully to
   what is said by all parties?   1   2   3   4   5

4. Does the interpreter share insights about
   a given culture in a manner that
   facilitates the process?   1   2   3   4   5

5. Does the interpreter appear to be respectful
   of both cultures and seem well respected by
   the community and the families that need
   the interpreter's services?   1   2   3   4   5

6. Is the interpreter willing to acquire new skills
   to perform the job more effectively? 1   2   3   4   5

7. Is there evidence that the interpreter
   maintains neutrality and confidentiality
   throughout the process?   1   2   3   4   5

8. Does the interpreter accept positive
   feedback from parents and other parties
   involved in the process?   1   2   3   4   5

9. Is the interpreter punctual?   1   2   3   4   5

Continued on next page

Figure 6.1—*Continued*

SPECIFIC INTERPRETATION/TRANSLATION SKILLS

1. Does the interpreter appear to convey
   a given message clearly?   1   2   3   4   5

2. Does the interpreter retranslate something
   when it is unclear to any participant
   during a session?   1   2   3   4   5

3. Does the interpreter use
   different methods of conveying the
   same information?   1   2   3   4   5

4. Does the interpreter appropriately use
   different levels of formality?   1   2   3   4   5

5. Does the translator appropriately use back translation
   to ensure that a given document has preserved its
   original meaning?   1   2   3   4   5

Garber and Mauffette-Leenders (1997). This assessment will need to be translated into the language used by the parent, relatives, or client, depending on the situation. If clients or family members have difficulty reading the survey, they could be encouraged to complete it at home with the help of a family member or friend.

Interpreters will need to be informed when hired that their performance evaluations will include feedback received from both the professionals working with them and clients. This feedback should be used only as part of the evaluation and is for the purpose of identifying areas of strength and areas that may need improvement. The survey results should not be the deciding factor in promoting or dismissing an interpreter. The

Consumer Evaluation
Figure 6.2 **of the Interpreter**

Dear _____,

Today you participated in a session where the services of an inter-preter, Mr./Ms. _____, were used. Your responses and feedback will help us monitor the quality of services provided by this person. Thank you for your time.

Language: _____

Date: _____

Purpose of the Session:

  To gather information   To share progress

To share assessment results   To assist with intervention

How many times have you worked with this interpreter?
$$1 \quad 2 \quad 3 \quad 4 \quad 5^+$$

How many times have you worked with this specialist? $1 \quad 2 \quad 3 \quad 4 \quad 5^+$

On a scale from 0 to 5, please rate the following questions:

    (0) Not applicable   (1) Very good   (2) Good
      (3) Average   (4) Below average   (5) Poor

1. How clearly did the communication disorders professional and the interpreter explain their roles to you?
$$0 \quad 1 \quad 2 \quad 3 \quad 4 \quad 5$$

2. How well did you understand this interpreter?
$$0 \quad 1 \quad 2 \quad 3 \quad 4 \quad 5$$

Continued on next page

  149

Figure 6.2—*Continued*

3. How accurately do you feel the interpreting was done?

   0 1 2 3 4 5

4. How assured do you feel that the information will be kept confidential?

   0 1 2 3 4 5

5. How well did you understand your rights regarding assessment, receiving a given procedure, or the therapy suggested?

   0 1 2 3 4 5

6. If you brought a bilingual advocate to the meeting, how well do you feel the team included this person's input?

   0 1 2 3 4 5

7. How well were your concerns or questions answered?

   0 1 2 3 4 5

8. Did the interpreter make you feel at ease?

   0 1 2 3 4 5

9. Please rate your satisfaction in working with an interpreter

   0 1 2 3 4 5

Please provide any further comments: _____

_____

_____

THANK YOU VERY MUCH FOR YOUR TIME.

From Obtaining Feedback from Non-English Speakers, by N. Garber and L.A. Mauffette-Leenders, In *The Critical Link: Interpreters in the Community* (pp. 131–143), by S.E. Carr, R. Roberts, A. Dufour, and D. Steyn (Eds.), 1997, Philadelphia: Johns Benjamins. © 1997 by Johns Benjamins. Adapted with permission.

assessment should be done in a constructive manner and based on several observations or situations.

Figure 6.3 (see pages 152–153) includes questions for an interpreter to complete to assess the effectiveness of the collaboration with a speech-language pathologist or audiologist. Interpreters can also use this form to evaluate themselves.

THE FUTURE OF INTERPRETERS IN SPEECH-LANGUAGE PATHOLOGY AND AUDIOLOGY

Even though the field of interpreting and translating has existed for a long time, it is hoped that further research on best practices will be conducted in the context of the collaboration that takes place between the interpreter and the speech-language pathologist or audiologist. Communication disorders professionals in all settings are encouraged to pursue investigations in these areas:

1. Conduct a survey to explore the current status of interpreter collaborations. Begin the survey in 10 states that have the highest numbers of CLD populations. Collect information regarding communication disorders professionals' number of experiences working with interpreters, types of interactions (e.g., conferences or assessments), knowledge base in the field of working with interpreters, and languages used.

2. Collect data on specific practices currently in use and document helpful strategies. Determine how many communication disorders professionals are familiar with the briefing, interaction, and debriefing (BID) process and how many communication disorders professionals follow this practice. Determine what the communication disorders professional's and the interpreter's roles are in the three steps. For example,

151

Figure 6.3   **Feedback from the Interpreter**

Setting: School   Clinic   Hospital

Date: _____

Length of conference: _____

Conference when the interpreting took place
      (please circle all that apply):
      To gather information   Assessment report

          Progress report   To assist with interpretation

How many times have you worked with this communication
      disorders professional?   1   2   3   4   5+

When do you work with this communication disorders professional?
      (circle all that apply):
      Interviews   Assessments   Assessments to report results
                  Progress reports   Intervention sessions

      Which are most frequent? _____

What type of interpreting do you typically use when working with
      a communication disorders professional?
      (Please circle all that apply):
            Consecutive   Simultaneous (or whispered)

Do you have time to brief and debrief with the communication
      disorders professional?   Y   N
If no, please state the reason(s) _____
If yes, how often:
      Almost always   Often   Sometimes   Rarely

1. Were you able to let the speech-language pathologist or audiol-
      ogist know that you did not agree with what he/she said after
      the meeting with the client?   Y   N

2. What suggestions do you have to improve service delivery
      when an interpreter is involved? _____
      _____

3. What are some of your personal reactions to the interpreter/
      communication disorders professional process? _____
      _____
      _____

Figure 6.3—*Continued*

4. What characteristics do you observe in a "good" communication disorders professional?_____

_____

5. What characteristics have you observed in a "poor" communication disorders professional?_____

_____

6. Any other comments?_____

_____

Interpreter Self-Assessment

Have you received any training for being an interpreter?　Y　N
If yes, where, when, and how long was the training?

_____

Have you taken any continuing education in this area?　Y　N
If yes, please describe: _____

On a scale from 0 to 5 please rate the following:

(0) Not applicable　　(1) Very good　　(2) Good
(3) Average　　(4) Below average　　(5) Poor

1. The accuracy of your interpreting was:　0　1　2　3　4　5

2. Your ability to keep information
confidential was:　　　　　　　　　0　1　2　3　4　5

3. Your ability to avoid giving direct advice to the client without the involvement of the communication disorders professional was:

0　1　2　3　4　5

4. Your ability to help the client understand his or her rights regarding assessment, why he or she was receiving a given procedure, or the nature of the therapy or intervention suggested was:　　　　　　0　1　2　3　4　5

5. If the client brought a bilingual advocate to the meeting, your ability to work collaboratively with that person was:

0　1　2　3　4　5

Source: Fradd (1993)

determine what the communication disorders professional's roles are during assessment. Also, determine the
indicators of a good and a poor performance by an interpreter in the eyes of a speech-language pathologist or
audiologist.

3. Survey interpreters in the field of speech-language
pathology and audiology. Have them describe their
training, daily practice, and the working conditions they
need to successfully fulfill their professional duties.

4. Survey clients who have received services from an
interpreter. Use questionnaires (such as Figure 6.2) to
determine indicators of good and poor interpreter performance from the client's point of view.

5. Identify specific strategies for working with interpreters in different settings (e.g., schools, clinics, hospitals, and agencies). Compare how the BID process is
carried out in different settings, and determine if the
process differs according to the age of the client or type
of communication disorder.

6. Compare and contrast practices in speech-language
pathology and audiology. This study would survey
practices used by each type of clinician regarding the
BID process. Comparisons across work settings would
yield information regarding whether certain steps are
more often omitted than others. For example, do most
audiologists brief with their interpreter, and do audiologists use the services of an interpreter more often for
conferences as compared to assessments?

7. Compare and contrast practices used in other fields of interpreting to refine best practices in working with speech-language pathologists and audiologists. Conduct a large-scale survey to define how the BID process is implemented by various disciplines. For example, what specific skills are needed in an interpreter working with a psychologist as compared with a special education teacher or a speech-language pathologist?

> Offer professional development opportunities to interpreters and the communication disorders professionals working with them.

8. Create preparation programs that will enable interpreters to be certified and recognized for the work they do. Implement professional development programs as suggested in this chapter to give communication disorders professionals and interpreters a common framework of currently known best practices.

9. Offer professional development opportunities to interpreters and the communication disorders professionals working with them. Discuss and expand a given topic according to the needs of specific groups. For example, some interpreters may need more practice in administering specific tests and tasks and some speech-language pathologists may need more practice in watching the interpreter assess a client.

155

10. Create a bank of tasks in various languages that could be used by teams that are assessing a client in a given language. For example, make a CD-ROM with curriculum-based assessments for different age and grade levels to assess specific skills, such as general knowledge and the ability to follow directions, comprehend paragraphs of different lengths and complexities, make verbal associations, and read various types of paragraphs in the given language.

APPENDICES

DESCRIPTIONS OF THE TOP 10 LANGUAGES SPOKEN IN THE WORLD

A language family is a group of languages that have been proven to descend from a common ancestral language. Branches of families represent groups of languages with a more recent common ancestor.

Typology is the study of similarities and differences between various languages (e.g., the position of a question word within a sentence, whether and how subject-verb agreement is marked, and the maximum number of prefixes or suffixes that can occur together on a word). In Table A.1 (see page 160), the only typology feature addressed is the basic constituent order of a sentence (i.e., subject, verb, object [SVO] or subject, object, verb [SOV]).

Phonetic features were defined by Nicolosi, Harryman, and Krescheck (1996) as:

Vowels: Voiced speech sounds resulting from the unrestricted passage of the air stream through the mouth or nasal cavity without audible friction or stoppage.

Consonants: Conventional speech sounds made with or without vocal fold vibration (i.e., voiced or unvoiced) by certain successive contractions of the articulatory muscles that modify, interrupt, or obstruct the expired air stream so that its pressure is raised.

Tones: Syllables produced with a characteristic pitch that influences the meaning of a word.

Table A.1

Description of the Top 10 Languages Spoken in the World

Language	Family, Branch, and Subbranch	Countries or Regions with over 500,000 Speakers	Number of Speakers	Typology	Phonetic Features
Mandarin	SINO-TIBETAN Chinese Mandarin	China, Taiwan, Russia, United States, South Africa, United Kingdom, parts of South America	885,000,000	SVO, SOV	37 vowels 35 consonants 4 tones
Spanish	INDO-EUROPEAN Italic Romance	Spain, Mexico, Central and South America, Caribbean, United States, Philippines	332,000,000	SVO	5 vowels 18 consonants
English	INDO-EUROPEAN Germanic West Germanic	United Kingdom, United States, Canada, other former colonies	322,000,000	SVO	12 vowels 27 consonants
Bengali	INDO-EUROPEAN Indo-Iranian Indo-Aryan	Bangladesh, India	189,000,000	SOV	14 vowels 32 consonants
Hindi	INDO-EUROPEAN Indo-Iranian Indo-Aryan	India, Bangladesh, Mauritius, South Africa	182,000,000	SOV	17 vowels 42 consonants

Table A.1—*Continued*

Language	Family, Branch, and Subbranch	Countries or Regions with over 500,000 Speakers	Number of Speakers	Typology	Phonetic Features
Portuguese	INDO-EUROPEAN Italic Romance	Portugal, Brazil, France, Paraguay, South Africa	170,000,000	SVO	12 vowels 21 consonants
Russian	INDO-EUROPEAN Slavic East Slavic	Russia and former republics of USSR, Israel	170,000,000	SVO	5 vowels 21 consonants
Japanese	JAPANESE Japanese Independent	Japan, United States	125,000,000	SOV	5 vowels 20 consonants no consonant clusters
German	INDO-EUROPEAN Germanic West Germanic	Germany, Austria, Russia, Kazakhstan, Poland, Brazil, United States	98,000,000	SVO	15 vowels 23 consonants
Wu	SINO-TIBETAN Chinese Wu	China	77,175,000	SVO	9 vowels 26 consonants 7 tones

Sources: Campbell (1995); Grimes (1999); Katzner (1986); Ruhen (1976)

TESTS IN LANGUAGES OTHER THAN ENGLISH

Aprenda: La Prueba de Logros en Español, Segunda Edición (1997)*
Author: Psychological Corporation
Psychological Corporation
555 Academic Court • San Antonio, TX 78204
Assesses various academic areas in grades K–8. Normed on a nationwide sample of Spanish–speaking students.

Arabic Language Screening Tests: Preschool and School-Age (1999)*
Authors: El-Halees, Y., and Wiig, E.
Schema Press
7101 Lake Powell Drive • Arlington, TX 76016
Tests development and delays in children's acquisition of Arabic for preschool (ages 3–6 years) and school-age children (ages 7–13 years). Normed in Jordan and Palestine.

Arabic Expressive-Receptive Vocabulary Test (2000)*
Authors: El-Halees, Y., and Wiig, E.
Schema Press
7101 Lake Powell Drive • Arlington, TX 76016
Probes receptive and expressive Arabic vocabulary for ages 3–13. Normed in Jordan and Palestine.

Assessment of Phonological Processes–Spanish (APP–Spanish) (1986)*
Author: Hodson, B.W.

---

* This test includes norms. However, the consumer needs to read the manuals carefully because this test may have been normed on monolingual Spanish-speaking or other-language-speaking subjects or on specific bilingual subjects.

Los Amigos Research Associates
7035 Galewood • San Diego, CA 92120
Assesses articulation, with a focus on analysis of phonological processes, for ages 3 years and above. Not a translation from the English version.

Batería de Lenguaje Objectiva y Criterial (BLOC) (2000)*
Author: Puyuelo,. S.M.
Masson
Ronda General Mitre 149 • Barcelona, Spain
Tests morphology, syntax, semantics, and pragmatics for ages 5–14 years. Developed and normed in Spain on monolingual Spanish-speaking subjects.

**Bilingual Language Proficiency Questionnaire–
Spanish (1985)**
Authors: Mattes, L.J., and Santiago, G.
Academic Communication Associates
Publication Center, Dept. IN-20
P.O. Box 4279 • Oceanside, CA 92052-4279
Questionnaire gauges parents' views regarding their child's language development and performance.

Bilingual Language Proficiency Questionnaire–Vietnamese (1996)
Authors: Mattes, L.J., and Nguyen, L.
Academic Communication Associates
Publication Center, Dept. IN-20
P.O. Box 4279 • Oceanside, CA 92052-4279
Questionnaire gauges parents views regarding their child's language development and performance.

---

* This test includes norms. However, the consumer needs to read the manuals carefully because this test may have been normed on monolingual Spanish-speaking or other-language-speaking subjects or on specific bilingual subjects.

Bilingual Syntax Measure (BSM) (1980)*
Authors: Burt, M.K., Dulay, H.C., Hernández-Chávez, E., and Taleporos, E.
Psychological Corporation
555 Academic Court • San Antonio, TX 78204
Tests oral language proficiency based on correct production of Spanish and English grammatical structures for grades K–2 (Level I) and grades 3 and above (Level II). Normed on a non-randomized group of Spanish-English bilingual speakers.

Bilingual Verbal Ability Test (1998)*
Authors: Muñoz-Sandoval, A.F., Cummins, J. Alvarado, C.G., and Ruef, M.L.
Riverside Publishing
425 Spring Lake Drive • Itasca, IL 60143-9921
Tests picture vocabulary, oral vocabulary, and verbal analogies in English and 16 other languages, including Arabic, two forms of Chinese, French, German, Haitian-Creole, Hindi, Italian, Japanese, Korean, Polish, Portuguese, Russian, Spanish, Turkish, and Vietnamese for grades K–12. Normed on a multilingual group.

Bilingual Vocabulary Assessment Measure (1995)
Author: Mattes, L.J.
Academic Communication Associates
Publication Center, Dept. IN-20
P.O. Box 4279 • Oceanside, CA 92052-4279
Screens for basic vocabulary in English, Spanish, French, Italian, and Vietnamese for ages 3 and up. This test is criterion referenced.

---

* This test includes norms. However, the consumer needs to read the manuals carefully because this test may have been normed on monolingual Spanish-speaking or other-language-speaking subjects or on specific bilingual subjects.

Boston Diagnostic Aphasia Examination–Revised (Spanish edition) published in *Evaluación de la Afasia y de Trastomos Relacionados* (1996)
Authors: Goodglass, H., and Kaplan, E.
Editorial Medica Panamericana
Buenos Aires, Argentina
Diagnoses types of aphasia and related disabilities in adults.

Bracken Basic Concept Scale (Revised)
Author: Bracken, B.A.
Psychological Corporation
555 Academic Court • San Antonio, TX 78204
Tests 11 concept categories (e.g., colors, letters, comparisons, directions, and textures/materials) for ages 2:6 to 7:11. A criterion referenced Spanish translation. Adaptations from the English version were made based on results from a small sample of Spanish-speaking children in the United States.

Clinical Evaluation of Language Fundamentals–3 (CELF–3) (Spanish edition) (1995)*
Authors: Semel, E., Wiig, E.H., and Secord, W.A.
Psychological Corporation
555 Academic Court • San Antonio, TX 78204
Assesses various aspects of language comprehension and expression for ages 6–21 years. Normed on bilingual subjects from the United States.

Cuaderno de Logoaudiometria (1994)
Authors: Cardenas, M., and Marrero, V.
Cuadernos de la UNGD

---

* This test includes norms. However, the consumer needs to read the manuals carefully because this test may have been normed on monolingual Spanish-speaking or other-language-speaking subjects or on specific bilingual subjects.

Universidad Nationale de Educación a Distancia • Madrid, Spain
Includes a CD-ROM that enables the assessor to evaluate auditory reception, discrimination, distinctive features, and central processing skills. This test can be used with all ages.

Dislexias y Disgrafias: Teoría, Formas Clínicas y Exploración (1998)
Authors: Lecours, A.R., Peña-Casanova, J., and Dieguez-Vide, F.
Masson
Ronda General Mitre 149 • Barcelona, Spain
Tests skills such as dictation, dictation of individual letters, oral comprehension, and other related tasks. This test, developed in Spain, can be used with all ages.

Dos Amigos Verbal Language Scales (DAVLS) (1996)
Author: Critchlow, D.E.
Academic Communication Associates
Publication Center, Dept. IN-20
P.O. Box 4279 • Oceanside, CA 92052-4279
Screens for language dominance and proficiency based on ability to provide opposites of various words in English and Spanish for ages 5–13 years. This test is criterion referenced.

Expressive One Word Picture Vocabulary Test (EOWPVT) Spanish-Bilingual Edition (2000)*
Author: Brownell, R.
Riverside Publishing
425 Spring Lake Drive • Itasca, IL 60143-9921
Tests ability to name words of increasing complexity. Normed on a national sample of bilingual Spanish people ages 4–12.

* This test includes norms. However, the consumer needs to read the manuals carefully because this test may have been normed on monolingual Spanish-speaking or other-language-speaking subjects or on specific bilingual subjects.

Fundación MacArthur Inventario del Desarrollo de Habilidades Comunicativas: Palabras y Enunciados (Spanish adaptation of the MacArthur Communicative Development Inventories) (1992)

Author: Fenson, L.

Department of Psychology

San Diego State University

5500 Campanile Drive • San Diego, CA 92182

Uses parent reports to test receptive and expressive vocabulary at 2 levels: infant and toddler.

IDEA Oral Language Proficiency Test, Spanish Version (1989)*

Author: Dalton, E.

Ballard and Tighe

P.O. Box 219 • Brea, CA 92822-0219

Tests language proficiency on several discrete language tasks for ages 3–5 years (Level 1), elementary (Level 2), and junior and senior high (Level 3).

Language Assessment Scales (1990)*

Authors: DeAvila, E., and Duncan, S.

McGraw-Hill

1221 Avenue of the Americas • New York, NY 10020

Tests Spanish language proficiency on several discrete language tasks for preschool (Pre–LAS), elementary (Level I), and secondary (Level II) levels. Normed on students in Mexico and southwest United States of mixed Spanish-English language backgrounds.

---

* This test includes norms. However, the consumer needs to read the manuals carefully because this test may have been normed on monolingual Spanish-speaking or other-language-speaking subjects or on specific bilingual subjects.

Medida Española de Articulación (MEDA) (1976)

Authors: Masson, M.A, Smith, B.F., and Hinshaw, M.M.

San Ysidro School District

2250 Smyth Avenue • San Ysidro, CA 92173

Measures articulation skills in Spanish using single words elicited with pictures in children ages 4–9 years of age.

Preschool Language Scale–3 (PLS–3) (Spanish version) (1992)*

Authors: Zimmerman, I.L., Steiner, V.G., and Pond, R.E.

Psychological Corporation

555 Academic Court • San Antonio, TX 78204

Assesses receptive and expressive language for ages birth to 6:11. Norms are available but must be interpreted carefully because they were performed only on specific items. A revision is in development.

Programa Integrado de Exploración Neurológica (1990)

Author: Peña, J.

Masson

Ronda General Mitre 149 • Barcelona, Spain

Assesses various neurologically based patterns, including spontaneous language, orientation, digits, reading, sequential use of objects, visual memory, and information. Developed in Spain.

---

* This test includes norms. However, the consumer needs to read the manuals carefully because this test may have been normed on monolingual Spanish-speaking or other-language-speaking subjects or on specific bilingual subjects.

Protocolo para la Valoración de la Audición y el Lenguaje en Lengua Español en un Programa de Implantes Cocleares (1996)

Authors: Huarte, A., Molina, M., Manrique, M., Olletta, J. García-Tapia, R.

Masson

Ronda General Mitre 149 • Barcelona, Spain

Assesses various audiological and linguistic aspects of pre- and postoperative candidates for cochlear implants. Includes areas such as pure tones, identification of vowels and consonants, monosyllabic and bisyllabic words, lip reading, voice, and articulation skills.

Pruebas de Expresión Oral y Percepción de la Lengua Española (PEOPLE) (1980)*

Los Angeles County Office of Education

9300 E. Imperial Highway • Downey, CA 90242

Tests discrete skills, such as auditory memory, auditory association, sentence repetition, encoding, and story comprehension, for ages 6:0 to 9:11 to identify children of Mexican descent who have a language disability. Normed on grade K–5 students in southern California.

Receptive One-Word Picture Vocabulary Test: Spanish-Bilingual Edition (ROWPVT–SBE) (2001)*

Author: Brownell, R.

Riverside Publishing

425 Spring Lake Drive • Itasca, IL 60143-9921

Tests vocabulary in children ages 2 through 12 who are

---

* This test includes norms. However, the consumer needs to read the manuals carefully because this test may have been normed on monolingual Spanish-speaking or other-language-speaking subjects or on specific bilingual subjects.

Spanish-English bilingual. Normed on national sample of bilingual speakers.

**Sequenced Inventory of Communication
Development–Spanish Translation (1984)**
Authors: Hedrick, D.L., Prather, E.M., and Tobin, A.R.
University of Washington Press
P.O. Box 50096 • Seattle, WA 98145
Assesses receptive and expressive language for children at developmental ages of 4 months to 4 years. This is a direct translation of the English version to Cuban Spanish.

Spanish Articulation Measures (Revised Edition) (1995)
Author: Mattes, L.J.
Academic Communication Associates
Publication Center, Dept. IN-20
P.O. Box 4279 • Oceanside, CA 92052-4279
Assesses 18 phonological processes through stimulability, spontaneous word production, and conversation for ages 3 years and above. Field tested in California bilingual education programs.

**Spanish Language Assessment Procedures (SLAP) (Third
Edition) (1995)**
Author: Mattes, L.J.
Academic Communication Associates
Publication Center, Dept. IN-20
P.O. Box 4279 • Oceanside, CA 92052-4279
Tests pragmatic and structural aspects of the Spanish language for ages 3–9 years. The test is criterion referenced.

**Spanish Test for Assessment of Morphologic Production
(STAMP) (1991)**
Authors: Nugent, T.M., Shipley, K.G., and Provencio, P.O.
Academic Communication Associates

Publication Center, Dept. IN-20

P.O. Box 4279 • Oceanside, CA 92052-4279

Assesses production of various Spanish morphemes following a developmental model for ages 5–11 years. May be used with a variety of Spanish dialects.

Structured Photographic Expressive Language Test–Spanish (1989)

Authors: Werner, E.O., and Kresheck, J.D.

Janelle Publications

P.O. Box 811 • Dekalb, IL 60115

Tests production of grammatical structures elicited with photographs for ages 3–5 years (Level I) and ages 5–8 years (Level II). The test does not follow a developmental model of Spanish language development. The test is criterion referenced.

Test de Vocabulario en Imágenes Peabody: Adaptación Hispanoamericana (TVIP) (1986)*

Authors: Dunn, L.M., Padilla, E.R., Lugo, D.E., and Dunn, L.M.

American Guidance Service

4201 Woodland Road • Circle Pines, MN 55014

Tests receptive vocabulary for ages 2:6 to 18:0 following the same model as the Peabody Picture Vocabulary Test. Normed on monolingual Spanish speakers in Mexico and Puerto Rico.

Test of Auditory Perceptual Skills–Revised, Spanish Version (1996)*

Author: Gardner, M.F.

Psychological and Educational Publishers

P.O. Box 520 • Hydesville, CA 95547–0520

Tests various auditory–based tasks such as discrimination, memory, and processing in subjects ages 5–13.

---

* This test includes norms. However, the consumer needs to read the manuals carefully because this test may have been normed on monolingual Spanish-speaking or other-language-speaking subjects or on specific bilingual subjects.

Woodcock Language Proficiency Battery–Revised (WLPB–R) (1995)*

Authors: Woodcock, R.W., and Muñoz-Sandoval, A.E.

Riverside Publishing

425 Spring Lake Drive • Itasca, IL 60143-9921

Tests the general level of language skills in English or Spanish for ages 4–adult. Normed on monolingual Spanish speakers in various countries, including the United States.

Woodcock-Muñoz Language Survey (WMLS) (2001)*

Authors: Woodcock, R.W., and Muñoz-Sandoval, A.F.

Riverside Publishing

425 Spring Lake Drive • Itasca, IL 60143-9921

Measures cognitive academic language proficiency in English and Spanish for ages 4–adult. Normed on a group matched to United States population characteristics.

---

* This test includes norms. However, the consumer needs to read the manuals carefully because this test may have been normed on monolingual Spanish-speaking or other-language-speaking subjects or on specific bilingual subjects.

CASE STUDIES

Arturo: A Spanish-Speaking 9 Year Old

Arturo's case illustrates the involvement of an interpreter during the phase of collecting information to understand his background and his parents' perceptions of his academic difficulties. This case uses the review, interview, observe, and test (RIOT) process. The speech-language pathologist and the interpreter also follow the briefing, interaction, and debriefing (BID) process in their collaborative planning and assessment of Arturo. In addition, this case explores the dynamics of the IEP meeting where the results and recommendations of the assessment were shared with the family.

Review

Arturo, age 9, was attending a bilingual third grade. He was referred for assessment because of academic difficulties, primarily reading comprehension problems in his primary language, Spanish. Additional concerns centered around his inability to express complex ideas in Spanish. Progress in English had been fair as reported by his classroom teachers.

Arturo received extensive assistance from a Spanish-speaking tutor, and his teacher spent extra time assisting him after school. Arturo made some progress over time, but his performance continued to be low compared with other bilingual students enrolled in the school. Arturo's teacher noticed that he did not participate very much in class, even when the interaction was in Spanish. He was quiet and he responded only when asked a question. He had friends and he liked to chat, but his verbal participation was limited. The district did not have a bilingual Spanish-English speech-language pathologist on staff.

Interview

The speech-language pathologist interviewed Arturo's parents with the help of the interpreter. They were very supportive of his education, even though they had not had an opportunity to attend formal school beyond sixth grade. They were enrolled in English classes, but their expressive English-language proficiency continued to be limited.

Arturo emigrated with his parents from Guatemala in the middle of his kindergarten year, which was his first opportunity to attend school. Arturo's health history was unremarkable, except that his speech developed later than that of his only sibling and other children in the community. Arturo's younger brother was progressing well in school, and no problems were observed in his use of either Spanish or English. Arturo was enrolled in the same type of bilingual program as his brother—a transitional program where instruction in Spanish was offered until third grade. His attendance was very good.

Arturo liked to watch TV and to ride his bike. He enjoyed following his father around the house and helping him fix anything from the car to a leaky faucet. Arturo had limited opportunities to play with others except for his brother or family friends who visited on weekends. His parents did not allow their children to play outside, because the apartment complex was near a busy street. On weekends the family enjoyed going to the park when the weather was good or visiting relatives and friends. Although Arturo liked to listen to oral and written stories that were read to him, his parents reported that he had a difficult time retaining the information. When they asked him questions about the story, he could not remember many facts.

Observation

The speech-language pathologist observed Arturo in his third-grade classroom. Arturo listened intently and tried to do his best, but he needed to ask his partner for help with oral and written directions. Classroom observation by the interpreter indicated that Arturo had fairly good basic communication skills in Spanish, but he did not initiate conversations with either peers or adults. He conversed about daily topics, such as his experiences and his preferences, but he had much more difficulty when he was asked to retell the plot of a story that the teacher had read in class. He decoded simple texts at the first-grade level, which was two years behind his current grade level. He solved a two-step math word problem. Unlike his classmates, he had not transitioned into using English in the classroom.

A recess observation by the interpreter indicated that Arturo was rather quiet. He preferred mingling with classmates who spoke Spanish to him. He did not initiate much of the interaction and his responses were brief.

The speech-language pathologist confirmed that several attempts to support Arturo's needs had been made by classroom staff. Arturo's teacher made a referral for a special education evaluation and explained it to Arturo's parents. They agreed to the assessment and gave their written consent to continue the process.

Testing

Briefing

The speech-language pathologist and interpreter met to review Arturo's case one day prior to the assessment. Both had already observed Arturo in the classroom and on the playground. The speech-language pathologist shared Arturo's portfolio and the transcription of his English narrative using *One Frog Too Many* (Mayer and Mayer, 1975), a wordless book. The speech-language pathologist commented that Arturo could convey some main ideas from the story, but the rendition of the story was very labored. Most of his narrative consisted of enumerating events, and it was up to the listener to interpret how the events were related. Arturo occasionally described how the characters felt and how they interacted, but the listener had to pay close attention to understand the essence of the story.

The speech-language pathologist was fortunate because the interpreter had already received extensive training through the County Office of Education and had worked closely with several speech-language pathologists in the previous two years. The interpreter was familiar with the process of assessment, and had been trained in the use of several testing materials available in Spanish. Nevertheless, the speech-language pathologist reviewed the assessment materials to make certain that the interpreter was familiar with them. The speech-language pathologist and the interpreter decided that Arturo would be given several subtests of the Spanish version of the Clinical Evaluation of Language Fundamentals–3 (CELF–3) (Wiig, Secord, and Semel, 1997) and the Test de Vocabulario en Imágenes Peabody (TVIP) (Dunn, Padilla, Lugo, and Dunn,

1986). They would ask him to narrate the same wordless book (*One Frog Too Many*) in Spanish. To encourage more verbalization, the speech-language pathologist and the interpreter decided that Arturo would invite his best friend to listen to his narrative of the wordless book.

They also planned to ask Arturo to complete the "Reading Comprehension" subtest of the Spanish version of the Brigance Diagnostic Assessment of Basic Skills (Brigance, 1983) to assess his ability to read paragraphs and answer questions. The speech-language pathologist would determine which modifications in test or task presentations would be needed to enhance his performance once the regular administration procedure had been implemented. The speech-language pathologist and interpreter planned to audiotape the interaction to review Arturo's answers and comments later as needed.

Interaction

The speech-language pathologist and the interpreter met Arturo together the same day as their briefing to prepare him for the testing. They explained their roles and indicated that the two of them would work with him at the same time because the interpreter would assist the speech-language pathologist to understand what Arturo would say in Spanish.

The next day, the speech-language pathologist and interpreter carried out the assessment. The speech-language pathologist was present during the entire testing time, which lasted 90 minutes with one 10-minute break. Arturo was cooperative, but he did not initiate very much of the conversation. He was somewhat more talkative when his friend visited to listen to his narrative. His rendition of the story *One Frog Too Many* (Mayer and Mayer, 1975) consisted of describing the pictures. The listener needed to pay close attention to understand the relationships between the characters in the story. Overall, Arturo tried his best, even though some of the tasks were difficult for him, especially when he had to respond to questions based on information presented in the form of stories, as on one of the CELF–3 Spanish subtests. It took him longer to respond than would be expected, and his answers were often incorrect.

The speech-language pathologist and the interpreter discussed how to enhance Arturo's responses. Using informal tasks, they observed that he was more accurate when the information was read more slowly and when it was stated a second time. Asking him to visualize the information was also helpful in enhancing his retention of the material presented.

Arturo had less difficulty on the "Formulating Sentences" subtest of the CELF–3, a task where he was asked to make up sentences in Spanish using the pictures and words provided. His short-term memory was weak when asked to repeat sentences of various lengths and complexities on the "Sentence Repetition" subtest of the CELF–3 (Spanish).

Arturo's reading in Spanish was labored at the second-grade level. Several miscues were noted and he was unable to answer comprehension questions based on the material he had read. Comprehension skills were better during silent reading as compared to oral reading, but Arturo could answer only two of the five questions. While Arturo was responding, both the speech-language pathologist and the interpreter took notes about the manner in which he was responding, and the interpreter wrote down all Arturo's responses verbatim.

Debriefing

The speech-language pathologist and the interpreter reviewed all the responses and data obtained from the assessment. They speculated that because Arturo had been introduced to them the day before the assessment, he felt less intimidated and apprehensive about the experience. Observations indicated that his cooperation was good and he seemed at ease. He smiled when he was praised for his effort. They also discussed the initial observations made during the screening in English so they could be included as part of the speech-language pathologist's assessment report. Arturo's difficulty in comprehending what he read was related to his difficulty in decoding specific words, mostly multisyllabic words, and reflected some of the challenges he had in processing auditory information. Overall, Arturo could express basic ideas in Spanish, but he had difficulty explaining more elaborate thoughts.

Based on Arturo's parents' report, school history, observations, and his performance on various tasks in both English and Spanish, the speech-language pathologist concluded that Arturo's learning problem was not related to the simultaneous acquisition of two languages. The problem reflected a language-processing difficulty in both Spanish and English.

IEP Process

The IEP meeting was attended by Arturo's parents, his classroom teacher, and a bilingual family member. The participants, with the assistance of the interpreter, explained the roles of the IEP team members and then interpreted the findings and recommendations from the assessment. The bilingual family member participated and asked questions that were interpreted back and forth by the interpreter. Even though the bilingual family member was present, the interpreter was responsible for interpreting all the information that was conveyed. After discussing the results of the assessment, the IEP team determined that Arturo would qualify for special education because of a speech-language disability. This decision was not based on test scores alone, but was supported by his performance on the modified test tasks, teacher and parent observations, and reports of his progress over time. The IEP team determined that because Arturo had difficulty in both languages and he was enrolled in a bilingual program, it would be best if the speech-language pathologist worked with him in English and consulted with his teacher on how to best work with him in the bilingual classroom using the same learning strategies. His tutor would also participate in the implementation of the IEP.

Arturo's parents were given suggestions on how to help him at home, such as providing examples and situations where he could practice expressing himself with greater elaboration in Spanish (e.g., explaining how to solve a given problem or how to fix his bike). The IEP team also recommended that Arturo receive additional reading instruction from a resource specialist. The team was optimistic that Arturo's cooperation, desire to improve, and parents' support would be great assets in enhancing his progress.

The interpreter, under the guidance of the speech-language pathologist, contacted the parents one week following their attendance at the IEP team meeting to ascertain if they had any further questions or concerns about the program and the recommendations. The interpreter reported that Arturo's parents were satisfied and they had already begun to implement some of the suggestions that had been provided during the meeting. They indicated that they were trying to give Arturo only a few directions, allowing more time for him to respond, and expanding on his ideas.

David: A Mandarin-Speaking 5 Year Old

David's case illustrates the need for additional time on the part of the speech-language pathologist and interpreter to ensure that the assessment is conducted fairly and that the parents understand the results and follow-up recommendations. These factors are often not taken into account.

David's case also illustrates the need to clearly identify the language spoken by the client so appropriate interpreter services can be located. Chinese is a family of mutually unintelligible languages, making it important to clearly identify the dialect before locating an interpreter. In this case, David's family spoke Mandarin, which is the literary standard in China but is unintelligible to speakers of other Chinese languages (e.g., Cantonese).

The interpreter assisted in gathering information about David's language development and his use of Mandarin and English. In contrast to Arturo, where initially it was not clear if he had a language disorder, David experienced significant problems that were evident in both Mandarin and English. Due to the lack of normed language tests in Mandarin, the speech-language pathologist needed to ensure that adequate information was collected. No norms could be used. The diagnosis and intervention were based on David's responses to informal measures, adapted items from a preschool test, and a language sample. Furthermore, this case was complicated because David's parents were anxious about his problem, had many questions about the etiology of the problem, and were seeking guidance on how to help David. The speech-language pathologist and the interpreter needed to take additional time to ensure that the parents' questions were answered and that the interpreter remained neutral and objective during the process.

Review

David was referred for an evaluation because of speech-language and behavioral concerns. When he was 2 years old, David could only say "mama" and "daddy" in Mandarin. His parents lived in Seattle until he was 3 years old, then moved to Michigan. His father spoke Mandarin and English to David. His mother interacted with David in Mandarin only as her English was still limited. David had a history of recurrent ear infections that were controlled after undergoing a myringotomy when he was 2½ years old.

When David's family moved to Michigan, he was placed in a daycare where only English was spoken. David continued using mostly single words in both languages, combined with some gestures. Since David began responding with greater ease in English once the family moved to Michigan, his mother also began interacting with him more in English, despite her limited proficiency in the language. By age 5, improvement was noted in both languages, but David's performance was not on par in either compared with other children who were growing up in a bilingual environment.

David was an only child. He had no other children with whom to interact in Mandarin, except on a few occasions when his parents visited friends or his grandparents came from China to visit the family. David's language history is described in Table C.1.

Table C.1 **David's Language History**

Age	Residence	Home/School Language	Language Performance
0–3	Seattle	Chinese/N/A	Only two words
3–4	Michigan	Chinese/English	Gestures & single words
4–5	Michigan	Mixed/English	Delayed English & Chinese

Since the speech-language pathologist did not speak Mandarin, and David's mother still interacted with greater ease in Mandarin, collaboration with an interpreter was necessary.

Interview

Although David's parents' command of English was fairly good, they still preferred having assistance from an interpreter for interviews with teachers and medical personnel. They were not always sure they were able to understand everything that was said or whether they could be easily understood. David's parents indicated that Mandarin continued to be the most prevalent language used during family interactions. They stated that Mandarin had to be used at home.

His parents indicated that they recently noticed David using longer sentences in English, but they realized that he was quite behind compared to other children with similar bilingual backgrounds. They were open and agreeable to professionals' assistance, and they were very involved in David's school. David's father was a member of the parents' committee, and his mother helped in the classroom. Even though Mandarin was used for interaction in the home, David seemed to pay more attention when his parents read to him in English. He responded in English even when spoken to in Mandarin, but he tried to speak Mandarin with his grandparents who could not understand English. Grammatical errors were noted in both languages, and he often mixed the two languages within the same sentence more than would be expected of a child who has been exposed to two languages (in contrast to patterns of code switching discussed in Chapter 2).

David enjoyed playing with blocks, and he made some very creative constructions. He interacted with other children, but he often got into fights because he was unable to understand everything they said and could not express himself adequately. David's teacher reported that he had adjusted well to the preschool environment and that he had made progress, yet he was not performing on par with other children for whom English was a second language. She was unsure if David could succeed in a kindergarten class the following year.

Observation

The speech-language pathologist interviewed David's teachers and observed him in the classroom. David appeared to be a happy child at school, except in situations where he had to express himself verbally. He played for extended times in the block area, but he had difficulty interacting with other children. Sharing space and toys often resulted in a fight with another child. When David spoke English, it was often difficult to understand what he wanted to say. When his mother was present in the classroom one day, she had difficulty understanding what he wanted in Mandarin. At times, it appeared that David had more ideas than he could convey. He enjoyed the circle time and listened to the story read by the teacher with great attention. On one or two occasions, he adequately answered a question that related to remembering certain facts. His responses consisted of a mixture of gestures and short sentences. The team's decision was to have a more in-depth assessment.

Testing

Briefing

The speech-language pathologist and interpreter met a week before the evaluation to plan the assessment. The speech-language pathologist selected specific items from the comprehension section of the Preschool Language Scale–3 (PLS–3) (Zimmerman, Steiner, and Pond, 1993), which she asked the interpreter to translate ahead of time. The items included assessing comprehension of various concepts (e.g., beginning and end and half and whole) and ability to follow specific directions using pictures. In addition, the speech-language pathologist reviewed vocabulary words on the Expressive One-Word Picture Vocabulary Test (EOWPVT) (Gardner, 1983), which she asked the interpreter to translate into Mandarin, and she requested that the interpreter verify if those particular words were used in the home. The speech-language pathologist planned to administer a Mandarin version of the Ecological Questionnaire (Cheng, 1991) and would accept responses in either language. In addition, the speech-language pathologist reminded the interpreter to ask clarification questions if something was confusing.

Interaction

David seemed at ease and motivated while interacting with the two adults, perhaps because he had met the speech-language pathologist and the interpreter ahead of time both at home and in school. He enjoyed responding to the adapted comprehension questions on the PLS–3 (Zimmerman, Steiner, and Pond, 1993) in Mandarin. More difficulty was noted when he needed to name the pictures on the EOWPVT (Gardner, 1983). Group words such as *fruit, animals,* and *furniture* were difficult to elicit. He had no label for *hammer, nail,* or *wheel* in any language, despite having experience with the words. His parents reported that he had seen his father do repairs in the house and name the items. He also had several toy cars, and the word *wheel* was frequently used. His expressive language consisted of three- to four-word utterances in Mandarin. Several utterances contained grammatical errors and many grammatical structures that mixed Mandarin and English. Although this pattern is not unusual for many bilingual students, in David's case, it was evident that it reflected his significant word retrieval difficulty. It took him a long time to say what he wanted to say; several hesitations and pauses were observed. More gestures than words were often included in his utterances. His pronunciation was clear in both languages for single words, but his intelligibility decreased in connected speech.

Debriefing

The speech-language pathologist felt that it was evident from the interviews, observations, and testing that David had a language disorder. The interpreter noted that David's language was significantly delayed compared to other children in his community who had been exposed to both Mandarin and English. The interpreter indicated that David's parents seemed aware of his problems but they felt intimidated by the entire testing process.

IEP Process

The IEP team met to discuss the assessment results and agreed that David should receive speech and language services. Much of the meeting was spent helping David's parents understand his language-learning needs and giving them strategies to help support the IEP goals. David's parents were appreciative of the information presented, but indicated in both English and Mandarin (in greater detail) that they were confused about what it all meant. They were unsure if David's language difficulty was their fault and what they could do to help him. His parents were afraid that exposure to two languages may have been the primary reason for his language delay. The speech-language pathologist explained the nature of David's problem and the possibility that multiple ear infections might have contributed to his language delay, but that bilingualism was not the cause of David's problem.

The speech-language pathologist suggested that David's parents speak to him using the language in which they felt more comfortable, which was Mandarin. Even though David's language preference was English at this time, it did not mean that he was unable to understand Mandarin, as indicated by observation and responses during testing. Furthermore, the speech-language pathologist explained that speaking to him in English at home would not necessarily enhance his competence in the language. She pointed out that it was preferable to offer him an intact language model in Mandarin, since his parents were still more comfortable speaking in that language as compared to English. When David responded in English instead of Mandarin, they were encouraged to respond in Mandarin by rephrasing and expanding what David had said in English. To foster his Mandarin language, the parents were encouraged to enroll David in a Saturday Chinese school so that he could interact more with peers in Mandarin.

Because David's parents were eager to speak English to him, the speech-language pathologist explained that selecting specific times for speaking that language would be helpful in assisting David to gain skills in English. She indicated that she was basing her recommendations on literature that had reported on how children attain optimal skills in bilingual environments (Arnberg, 1987; Baker, 1995; Harding and Riley, 1986).

Throughout the interaction, the interpreter maintained the role of conveying accurate information. She needed to ensure that both verbal and nonverbal messages were clearly understood and that the parents understood what the speech-language pathologist was saying. This meant requesting clarification from the speech-language pathologist at any sign of confusion from the parents. To ensure that all information was clear, the speech-language pathologist suggested a follow-up meeting within two weeks.

Marta: A 68-Year-Old Spanish-Speaking Stroke Patient

In Arturo's and David's cases, the process included reviewing the information, interviewing the family, observing, and testing (RIOT). In the case of an individual who is admitted to the hospital because of a stroke or traumatic injury, a review of medical records and an interview of the patient or relatives may need to be done within a few hours of admission. Consequently, the process to follow will depend on the particular case. The type of lesion, the degree of trauma, the impact on the patient's general health, and neurological findings will dictate the assessment procedures and further recommendations. Therefore, there might be very limited time during which the speech-language pathologist and the interpreter can brief about the case. In this case, Marta's daughter was available to provide detailed information.

Review

The speech-language pathologist and the interpreter reviewed Marta's medical records prior to conducting an assessment. Marta, a 68-year-old monolingual Spanish-speaking patient, was admitted to the hospital following a stroke. The medical and neurological evaluation indicated that she had sustained a left hemispheric cerebrovascular accident (CVA) that had resulted in right hemiplegia.

Interview

An interview with Marta's daughter, whose preferred language was Spanish, revealed that Marta had been a fairly healthy woman. Although she was overweight for her height, she had not had any signs of heart disease, except for having sudden dizzy spells. A medical evaluation three months prior to her stroke indicated that her blood pressure was very high. Medical treatment and a weight control and exercise program had been recommended, but Marta did not follow the doctor's recommendations. On the morning of her 68th birthday, Marta got out of bed and fainted on the way to the bathroom. She was taken to the hospital by ambulance.

Marta was originally from Oaxaca, Mexico and had been living in the United States for about 10 years. In her native country, Marta came from a fairly well-established family and had completed high school. She was the owner of the only grocery store in the small town of Oaxaca and previously had been in the United States only two times for short visits. Her command of English was limited.

Observation

Due to the setting and circumstances, observation was not appropriate. The speech-language pathologist relied on Marta's daughter to provide a description of Marta's normal communication behaviors.

Testing

Briefing

The speech-language pathologist decided to administer portions of the Boston Diagnostic Aphasia Examination (Revised) (Goodglass and Kaplan, 1983), which is available in a Spanish edition. The interpreter was not familiar with the test, so the speech-language pathologist reviewed the directions and tasks with her and asked her to review it further before Marta's appointment.

Interaction

The interpreter needed close guidance during administration of the standardized test. The speech-language pathologist followed along on the equivalent English version of each subtest the interpreter administered. Both the interpreter and the speech-language pathologist wrote down Marta's responses to questions and descriptions of pictures. The speech-language pathologist made notations about what she observed in the patient and the manner in which the interpreter was relating Marta's answers. For example, notations were made if additional cues from the interpreter were helpful in gaining more oral responses from Marta.

Marta was able to understand questions and could communicate to a limited degree, so a brief interview was possible. Marta expressed some of her frustrations and her desire to go back to her daughter's home. The interpreter had to pay close attention to what Marta was saying because her speech was not very clear. The interpreter reliably recorded when Marta was unsure about a given response. The interpreter frequently asked the speech-language pathologist for ideas on how to proceed and transcribed Marta's conversational language sample as accurately as she could.

Debriefing

The speech-language pathologist and the interpreter had only a half hour to debrief. The speech-language pathologist's analysis of Marta's response patterns indicated a transcortical motor aphasia. Marta's expressive language was limited, with some intonation difficulties, dysarthria, and reduced use of certain forms like articles and prepositions. Marta understood what was said to her, she could repeat some of the target sentences, and her naming skills were intact. The speech-language pathologist and the interpreter used their debriefing time to plan the follow-up conference.

Family Conference

During the follow-up conference with Marta and her family, the speech-language pathologist explained the results of the testing. She indicated that part of therapy would consist of helping Marta understand the nature of her communication problem and develop strategies to compensate for her lack of fluency. The interpreter and the speech-language pathologist would collaborate on those strategies during Marta's stay in the hospital and would continue to see her as an outpatient. The speech-language pathologist indicated that, given Marta's medical condition and the profile that was observed, her speech would likely improve within the next three months. However, the course of improvement was difficult to predict since it varies from patient to patient. If Marta continued to feel frustrated, counseling might be necessary. Marta had made friends with the priest in her church and he was willing to support her recovery. Plans were made to ask him to come the following week for the medical follow-up and a speech and language reevaluation conference.

Marta remained in the hospital for one week. The medical follow-up indicated a continued mild hemiplegia, which prevented her from walking without support from a cane. Her fluency had increased, but therapy for 30 minutes three times a week was recommended for up to six weeks. The priest and Marta's daughter volunteered to attend the sessions. Due to the scarcity of interpreters in the hospital, it was improbable that the interpreter could attend all the sessions. Therefore, during the therapy, the speech-language pathologist modeled strategies to increase fluency that were interpreted to Marta and used by Marta's daughter and the priest.

After six weeks, Marta's fluency and oral communication skills were close to normal, and her feelings of frustration and depression had subsided. Although she needed a cane to walk, Marta was happy to feel better. Because of her trauma, she lost close to 25 pounds and she vowed to continue on a diet and exercise plan. After being dismissed, Marta began taking long daily walks.

Marta's case had a happy ending. Not all cases have positive outcomes. A patient may progress more slowly, make some gains and then regress, or simply deteriorate. It is difficult enough for a patient who has sustained a traumatic injury to communicate in English. When, in addition, a language barrier separates patients from direct communication with clinicians and physicians, they can feel even more isolated. The availability and appropriate training of interpreters is therefore crucial. However, the limitations of health-care plans reduce the likelihood of hiring and training interpreters in this setting.

Every effort should be made to document the important job interpreters perform in the process of assessing and rehabilitating patients who have acquired a communication disorder.

Nguyen: A 74-Year-Old Vietnamese-Speaking Patient with a Hearing Problem

The case of Nguyen, a 74-year-old Vietnamese-speaking woman, illustrates the nature of an interpreter's involvement in an audiological evaluation. Because an interpreter was unavailable for the testing session, the briefing was carried out only after Nguyen's visit to the otolaryngologist.

Review

The audiologist obtained a chart with Nguyen's medical history, which seemed unremarkable except for the hearing complaint. Due to lack of available interpreters to assist her during the testing session, the audiologist proceeded to test Nguyen and hoped for reliable results.

Interview

Nguyen's son sent a note in English to the audiologist describing her complaints, which included not hearing him from a fairly close distance, needing to ask for repetition, and being annoyed if she could not hear in a restaurant where there was noise. Despite her lack of English, Nguyen could understand when the audiologist asked her which ear was causing the problem and how bad her hearing loss seemed to be.

Observation

Due to the clinical setting, an observation was not appropriate. The audiologist relied on interviews to determine how Nguyen's hearing was affecting her daily interactions.

Testing

All communication was conveyed with simple directions and many gestures. Nguyen could understand what she had to do when she heard a tone (i.e., raise her hand). The results of the audiogram indicated that she had a moderate hearing loss in her left ear and mild loss in her right ear. Nguyen was concerned about the reason for her hearing loss and communicated her question in broken English. The audiologist indicated through gestures and slow speech that she could not explain the reason for the loss, but that the otolaryngologist could give her a diagnosis. This was difficult for Nguyen to understand, but the audiologist's secretary set up an appointment with the otolaryngologist before Nguyen left the office. This helped Nguyen feel less anxious.

During her visit with the otolaryngologist, Nguyen found out that she had presbycusis and no other ear pathology. In the otolaryngologist's office, the physician and the interpreter explained the condition to her. A hearing aid was recommended to assist Nguyen's hearing acuity.

Follow-up Visit

Briefing

During her follow-up visit to the audiologist, the fitting and use of hearing aids were explained more directly to Nguyen because an interpreter was present. Prior to counseling Nguyen about the best hearing aids for her case, the audiologist and the interpreter had a short briefing time during which the audiologist summarized Nguyen's previous visit and concerns. Since the interpreter had been present at the otolaryngologist visit, he also had that background information on the hearing condition.

Interaction

Following the briefing, the audiologist and the interpreter were able to explain the range and type of hearing aid that would fit Nguyen's needs. Even though she was reluctant to wear any hearing aids, Nguyen agreed to try wearing the recommended hearing aid in her left ear. The presence of the interpreter had been helpful because Nguyen was able to express her embarrassment about her need to wear a hearing aid. She was unsure if it would help or if she could get used to it. The audiologist was able to answer Nguyen's questions and reassure her. An appointment to fit her hearing aid was scheduled.

Debriefing

The audiologist and the interpreter had some time to debrief after the session. They discussed the fact that if the interpreter had been present during the initial evaluation, Nguyen may have felt less anxious about her visit to the otolaryngologist and the need for her hearing aid. The interpreter indicated that, in his opinion, the presence of someone who can bridge the language barrier is important to make the patient more at ease. The audiologist decided to seek the assistance of an interpreter as much as possible in the future.

Summary

The RIOT procedure provided a useful framework for the communication disorders professional and interpreter collaborations. The following observations are common to most assessment situations:

• Interpreters participate in gathering and sharing information between professionals and people from different ages and educational backgrounds. Their intervention is needed in both speech-language pathology and audiology.

• Interpreters should be well prepared to conduct a fair assessment under the guidance of the speech-language pathologist or audiologist. Their participation is more critical in speech, language, and communication assessments as compared to audiological assessments because the entire assessment focuses on evaluating the client's receptive and expressive language skills. Ideally, however, interpreters should be present to assist both types of professionals in evaluations.

• Different procedures may be used when there are materials available in the primary language.

• Because audiological evaluations are more objective and require limited verbal responses from patients, interpreter participation in this phase of the assessment may not be as critical. Directions can be given with demonstrations and gestures that are universal in nature. However, a medical history assists in evaluating the patient accurately and can be collected more completely with the help of an interpreter. An audiologist might be able to evaluate the patient's hearing without an interpreter if a medical chart is available. If there is no medical information, the assistance of an inter-preter is needed to obtain the information.

- The assessment process demands specific preparation on the part of the speech-language pathologist or audiologist as well as the interpreter. The success of the process depends on their strong collaboration.

- Both speech-language pathologists and audiologists must understand the interpreting process and remember that inter-preters bridge communication between the professional and the family or the client. However, the ultimate diagnosis and path of intervention is always the responsibility of the speech-language pathologist or audiologist.

SAMPLE REPORT: BOPHA—A CAMBODIAN-SPEAKING PRESCHOOL CHILD

Reason for Referral

Bopha, age 4 years and 2 months, was referred by her Head Start teacher because of slow language development in English compared with other children who were learning English as a second language. She was not as verbal as other children who spoke Cambodian in her class.

History

Since Bopha's parents did not speak English, a parent interview was completed using the services of a trained Cambodian- and English-speaking interpreter from the school district.

Bopha's language development in Cambodian was similar to that of her siblings, and no problems were noted except for her pronunciation of certain words. Bopha was a healthy child with no hearing infections or health problems in her infancy. A hearing screening when she enrolled in preschool at age 3 years, 6 months was normal.

Bopha is the youngest of six children whose ages range from 4 to 18 years. Cambodian is spoken by the adults in the family, and both English and Cambodian are spoken by Bopha's siblings.

Assessment

The assessment consisted of observations, a normed test, and a language sample collected in various contexts. Similar areas were evaluated in both English and Cambodian.

Briefing

The Cambodian interpreter met and interacted with Bopha prior to the assessment during a home visit to obtain the signature of Bopha's mother on the assessment plan. The speech-language pathologist met with the interpreter the day before the testing session to plan the assessment. The speech-language pathologist reviewed her observations and Bopha's performance on the PLS–3 (Zimmerman, Steiner, and Pond, 1993) and language sample in English. The speech-language pathologist and the interpreter planned to readminister the difficult items from the PLS–3 using Cambodian. While reviewing the particular items that needed to be administered, the speech-language pathologist reminded the interpreter about the importance of enabling Bopha to respond without the need for additional cues such as gestures, intonation, or excessive repetitions. The speech-language pathologist and the interpreter agreed that if Bopha had difficulty responding to items the first time they were administered, different ways of facilitating her answers would be used to enhance her responses. However, this strategy would be used only after the interpreter and the speech-language pathologist had decided on the best method to follow. An audiotaped language sample would be obtained by inviting Bopha to play with the dollhouse.

Assessment in English

The speech-language pathologist observed and interacted with Bopha to examine her performance in English. The Preschool Language Scale–3 (PLS–3) (Zimmerman, Steiner, and Pond, 1993) was administered. A 75–utterance language sample was collected while Bopha played with the speech-language pathologist and a peer using a dollhouse (her favorite toy), other toys, and books.

Bopha's comprehension skills were commensurate with those of a younger child (2–3 years). Bopha followed simple instructions, but she was confused with prepositions like *in front* and *behind.* She recognized two colors consistently, and she pointed to several body parts. She had more difficulty pointing to finer body parts like *fingers, elbows,* or *knees* even though she had participated in numerous classroom activities involving touching knees, elbows, and toes as the class listened to songs. Bopha did not point to finer parts of objects or animals. She sorted pictures according to various categories.

Bopha's play skills were age appropriate but her verbalizations were minimal. While playing with dolls, Bopha pretended they were going to have a party. She set up a table with dishes and said "have cake," and at one point she said "ma go to" (mom going to the store). When the party was over, she pretended that the doll had to go to bed because "he ti" (she is tired). Bopha's expressive language included mostly two- or three-word combinations in English. She made several articulation errors, including omission of final /r/, /d/, /g/, /b/, and /z/. Voice, resonance, and an oral peripheral examination indicated no abnormalities in structure or function.

Assessment in Cambodian

The interpreter readministered items from the PLS–3 (Zimmerman, Steiner, and Pond, 1993) that Bopha had failed in English. The speech-language pathologist observed the entire session and asked for clarifications when it was unclear what the interpreter or Bopha had said. Since the tasks were receptive in nature, Bopha's expressive language output was minimal. There was a significant lag time between the interpreter's questions and Bopha's responses. On several occasions, the questions needed to be repeated and rephrased to obtain a response from Bopha. In other instances, the interpreter needed to ask Bopha to repeat what she had said. The interpreter reported that she could not understand Bopha very well because she was not pronouncing words very clearly. When Bopha imitated words modeled by the interpreter, her articulation improved but several errors were still noted. During the play session, the interpreter noted that Bopha was more talkative and responsive than

Debriefing

The interpreter made notes during the session (e.g., when she felt that Bopha had not understood a question). The interpreter also accurately transcribed what Bopha said without changing her words to the corrected forms. The speech-language pathologist and the interpreter reviewed these notes and the course of the assessment. To ensure that they had recorded all the data accurately, they played back the session audiotape to verify their observations.

she had been in English. Overall, Bopha was cooperative and she seemed to enjoy the individual attention.

Bopha responded with greater ease in Cambodian. Her comprehension skills and knowledge of concepts were approximately one year higher in Cambodian than in English (i.e., 3–4 years). Bopha processed information slowly and she needed extra time to respond. Her expressive language skills appeared more developed in Cambodian than in English. She used more complex linguistic structures, but it was difficult to understand her because she made numerous articulation errors. Because there are no data on language development in Cambodian, the interpreter relied on her experience with children of different ages. Her general impression was that Bopha sounded like a 3½-year-old child, primarily because of pronunciation problems.

Comparing Cambodian sounds (Cheng, 1991) with Bopha's current repertoire indicated that she could use most of the consonants in Cambodian except for /s/ and /d/. She had difficulty with sounds that exist in English but not in Cambodian, and with several sounds that are in different positions in words in English and Cambodian. Imitation of words in both languages was average, depending on the particular word.

Conclusions

Based on the observations provided by the parents and teachers, along with the assessment in both languages, Bopha appeared to qualify for special education services because of a speech and language impairment.

Recommendations

Goals should include improving Bopha's articulation skills and developing strategies for listening and processing. Therapy should be implemented in a small group for 30 minutes once a week and in the classroom for an additional 30 minutes per week.

Because of the lack of availability of an interpreter, intervention should take place in English. Bopha's parents can support her speech and language development in Cambodian with the following activities:

1. Name activities or items in Bopha's environment during conversation to develop her vocabulary.

2. Model the words that Bopha mispronounces by repeating them in a short phrase, but avoid correcting her and making her conscious of her errors.

3. Tell her stories and sing to her in Cambodian to further develop her language skills.

4. Use the language they are most fluent in to provide good language models for Bopha. (Children can develop two languages, so the family should not worry that they should speak only English to Bopha at home.)

Bopha's parents should conference with the speech-language pathologist and interpreter every other month to follow up on Bopha's progress.

REFERENCES

Aleksandrovsky, I.V., McCullough, J.K., and Wilson, R.H (1998). Development of a suprathreshold word recognition test for Russian-speaking patients. *Journal of the American Academy of Audiology, 9,* 417–425.

American Speech-Language-Hearing Association (1994). Code of ethics. *Asha, 40*(Suppl. 18), 43–45.

American Speech-Language-Hearing Association (ASHA) (1998). *Speech-language pathology assistants: Information Series.* Rockville, MD: Author. (Available from American Speech-Language-Hearing Association, 10801 Rockville Pike, Rockville, MD 20852)

Arnberg, L. (1987). *Raising children bilingually: The preschool years.* Clevedon, England: Multilingual Matters.

August, D., and Hakuta, K. (Eds.). (1998). *Educating language-minority children.* Washington, DC: National Research Council Institute of Medicine.

Australian Institute of Interpreters and Translators. (2000). *AUSIT Code of Ethics.* Retrieved May 25, 2001, from the World Wide Web: http://www.ausit.org/code.html

Baker, C. (1995). *A parents' and teachers' guide to bilingualism.* Clevedon, England: Multilingual Matters.

Baker, C., and Jones, S.P. (1998). *Encyclopedia of bilingualism and bilingual education.* Clevedon, England: Multilingual Matters.

Battle, D.E. (1993). *Communication disorders in multicultural populations.* Stoneham, MA: Butterworth-Heinemann.

Benmaman, V. (1997). Legal interpreting by any other name is still legal interpreting. In S.E. Carr, R. Roberts, A. Dufour, and D. Steyn (Eds.), *The critical link: Interpreters in the community* (pp. 179–190). Philadelphia: Johns Benjamins.

Bergman, C. (1976). Interference vs. independent development in infant bilingualism. In G. Keller, T. Teschner, and S. Viera (Eds). *Bilingualism in the bicentennial and beyond* (pp. 86–96). New York: Bilingual Press/La Revista Bilingue.

Berman, R., and Slobin, D. (1994). *Relating events in narrative: A crosslinguistic developmental study.* Hillsdale, NJ: Erlbaum.

Bracken, B.A., and McCallum, S.R. (2001). Assessing intelligence in a population that speaks more than two hundred languages: A nonverbal solution. In L.A. Suzuki, J.G. Ponterotto, and P.J. Miller (Eds.), *Handbook of multicultural assessment: Clinical, psychological, and educational applications* (2nd ed.) (pp. 405–431). San Francisco: Jossey-Bass.

Brigance, A. (1983). *Brigance diagnostic assessment of basic skills* (Spanish version). North Billerica, MA: Curriculum Associates.

Brislin, R.W. (1981). *Cross-cultural encounters: Face-to-face interaction.* New York: Pergamon.

Burgoon, J.K., Buller, D.B., and Woodall, W.G. (1996). *Nonverbal communication: The unspoken dialogue.* New York: McGraw-Hill.

Butler, K., and Cheng, L.L. (Eds.). (1996). Beyond bilingualism: Language acquisition and disorders—A global perspective [Issue]. *Topics in Language Disorders, 16(4).*

California Education Code, Title 5, Section 3023(a).

California State Department of Education (Ed.). (1991). _Towards a culturally competent system of care._ Sacramento, CA: Author.

California Speech-Language-Hearing Association. (1997). _Technical report on the utilization of speech aides in the public schools in California._ Sacramento, CA: Author.

California State Personnel Board (1998–2000). _Certification examination for medical interpreters_ [Information and application packet]. Sacramento, CA: Author.

Campbell, G.L. (1995). _Compendium of the world's languages._ London: Routledge.

Campbell, G.L. (1997). _Handbook of scripts and alphabets._ London: Routledge.

Cárdenas, M., and Marrero, V. (1994). _Cuaderno de logoaudiometría. Cuadernos de la UNED._ Madrid, Spain: Universidad Nacional de Educación a Distancia.

Carr, S.E. (1997). A three-tiered health care interpreter system. In S.E. Carr, R. Roberts, A. Dufour, and D. Steyn (Eds.), _The critical link: Interpreters in the community_ (pp. 271–276). Philadelphia: Johns Benjamins.

Cheng, L.L. (1989). Service delivery to Asian Pacific LED children: A cross-cultural framework. _Topics in Language Disorders, 9_(3), 1–14.

Cheng, L.L. (1990). The identification of communicative disorders in Asian-Pacific students. _Journal of Childhood Communication Disorders, 13_(1), 113–119.

Cheng, L.L. (1991). _Assessing Asian language performance_ (2nd ed.). Oceanside, CA: Academic Communication Associates.

Cheng, L.L. (1994a). Asian/Pacific students learning English. In J.E. Bernthal and N.W. Bankson (Eds.), _Child phonology:_

Characteristics, assessment and intervention with special popula-
tions (pp. 255–274). New York: Thieme Medical Publishers.

Cheng, L.L. (1994b). Difficult discourse: An untold Asian story.
In D.N. Ripich and N.A. Creaghead (Eds.), *School discourse*
problems (2nd ed.) (pp. 165–170). San Diego, CA: Singular.

Cheng, L.L. (1995). *Integrating language and learning for inclu-*
sion. San Diego, CA: Singular.

Cheng, L.L. (1996). Beyond bilingualism: A quest for communicative competence. *Topics in Language Disorders,16*(4),
9–21.

Cheng, L.L. (1998a). Beyond multiculturalism: Cultural translators make it happen. In V.O. Pang and L.L. Cheng (Eds.),
Struggling to be heard (pp. 105–122). Albany, NY: SUNY Press.

Cheng, L.L. (1998b, March). *Learning from multiple perspec-*
tives. Keynote address. at the ABC School District Annual
Parent Conference Los Angeles, CA.

Cheng, L.L. (1999). Moving beyond accent: Social and cultural
realities of living with many tongues. *Topics in Language*
Disorders, 19(4), 1–11.

Cheng, L., and Butler, K. (1989). Code-switching: A natural
phenomenon vs. language deficiency. *World Englishes,*
8(3), 293–310.

Cheng, L.L., Landgon, H.W., and Davies, D. (1991). *The art of inter-*
preting: A dynamic process. [Video]. San Diego, CA: Department
of Communication Disorders, San Diego State University.

Choi, S. (1997). Language-specific input and early semantic
development. In D.I. Slobin (Ed.), *The crosslinguistic student*
of language acquisition (pp. 41–133). Hillsdale, NJ: Erlbaum.

Comrie, B. (1992). Languages of the world. In W. Bright (Ed.), _International encyclopedia of linguistics_ (Vol. 2, pp. 305–310). New York: Oxford University Press.

Corsellis, A. (1997). Training needs of public personnel working with interpreters. In S.E. Carr, R. Roberts, A. Dufour, and D. Steyn (Eds.), _The critical link: Interpreters in the community_ (pp. 77–89). Philadelphia: Johns Benjamins.

Crystal, D. (1997). _The Cambridge encyclopedia of language_ (2nd ed.). New York: Cambridge University Press.

Cummins, J. (1984). _Bilingualism and special education._ Clevedon, England: Multilingual Matters.

Damico, J. (1991). Descriptive assessment of communicative ability in limited English proficiency students. In E.V. Hamayan and J.S. Damico (Eds.), _Limiting bias in the assessment of bilingual students_ (pp. 157–217). Austin, TX: Pro-Ed.

Diversity Rx. (1997). _Overview of role and practice issues._ Retrieved May 25, 2001, from the World Wide Web: http://www.diversityrx.org/html/moipri1.htm

Dunn, L.M., Padilla, E.R., Lugo, D.E., and Dunn, L.M. (1986). Test de Vocabulario en Imágenes Peabody (TVIP). Circle Pines, MN: American Guidance Service.

Edwards, J. (1994). _Multilingualism._ New York: Penguin Books.

Ekman, P. (1975, September). The universal smile: Face muscles talk every language. _Psychology Today, 9,_ 35–39.

El-Halees, Y., and Wiig, E.H. (1999). Arabic Language Screening Tests: Preschool and School Age. Arlington, TX: Schema Press.

El-Halees, Y., and Wiig, E.H. (2000). Arabic Receptive-Expressive Vocabulary Test. Arlington, TX: Schema Press.

Englund Dimitrova, B. (1997). Degree of interpreter responsibility in the interaction process in community interpreting.
In S.E. Carr, R. Roberts, A. Dufour, and D. Steyn (Eds.),
The critical link: Interpreters in the community (pp.
147–164). Philadelphia: Johns Benjamins.

Fadiman, A. (1997). *The spirit catches you and you fall down: A
Hmong child, her American doctors, and the collision of two
cultures.* New York: Farrar, Straus and Giroux.

Fishman, J.A. (1991) *Reversing language shift.* Clevedon,
England: Multilingual Matters.

Flege, J., and Bohn, O. (1989). An instrumental study of
vowel-reduction and stress placement in Spanish-accented
English. *Studies in Second Language Acquisition, 22,* 35–62.

Fleischman, J.L., and Hopstock, P.J. (1993). *Descriptive study of
services to limited English proficient students (Vol. 1):
Summary of findings and conclusions.* Arlington, VA:
Development Associates.

Flores, P., Martin, F.N., and Champlin, C.A. (1996). *American
Journal of Audiology, 5*(1), 69–73.

Fortier, J.P. (1997). Interpreting for health in the United States:
Government partnership with communities, interpreters
and providers. In S.E. Carr, R. Roberts, A. Dufour, and D.
Steyn (Eds.), *The critical link: Interpreters in the community*
(pp. 165–177). Philadelphia: Johns Benjamins.

Fowler, Y. (1997). The courtroom interpreter: Paragon and
intruder? In S.E. Carr, R. Roberts, A. Dufour, and D. Steyn
(Eds.), *The critical link: Interpreters in the community* (pp.
191–211). Philadelphia: Johns Benjamins.

Fradd, S.H. (1993). *Creating the team to assist culturally and linguistically diverse students.* Tucson, AZ: Communication Skill Builders.

Garber, N., and Mauffette-Leenders, L.A. (1997). Obtaining feedback from non-English speakers. In S.E. Carr, R. Roberts, A. Dufour, and D. Steyn (Eds.), *The critical link: Interpreters in the community* (pp. 131–143). Philadelphia: Johns Benjamins.

Garcia, E. (1991). *The education of linguistically and culturally diverse students: Effective instructional practices.* Washington, DC: National Center for Research for Cultural Diversity and Second Language Learning–Center for Applied Linguistics.

García-Albea, J., Sánchez, M., and Del Viso, S. (1982). Test de Boston para el diagnóstico de la afasia: Adaptación española. In H. Goodglass and E. Kaplan, *La evaluación de la afasia y transtornos asociados.* Buenos Aires, Argentina: Médica Panamericana.

Gardner, M.F. (1983). Expressive One-Word Language Test (Level 1). Novato, CA: Academic Therapy.

Gehrke, M. (1993). Community interpreting. In C. Picken (Ed.), *Translation: The vital link. Proceedings of the XIIIth World Congress of FIT* (Vol. 1). (pp. 417–421). London: Institute of Translation and Interpreting.

Gentile, A. (1997). Community interpreting or not? Practices, standards and accreditation. In S.E. Carr, R. Roberts, A. Dufour, and D. Steyn (Eds.), *The critical link: Interpreters in the community* (pp. 109–118). Philadelphia: Johns Benjamins.

Gersten, R.M., and Jiménez, R.T. (Eds.). (1998). *Promoting learning for culturally and linguistically diverse students.* Belmont, CA: Wadsworth.

Gerver, D., and Sinaiko, H.W. (Eds.). (1977). *Language interpretation and communication.* New York: Plenum Press.

Gile, D. (1986). La reconnaissance des kango et la perception du discours japonais. *Lingua, 70*(2/3), 171–189.

Gile, D. (1995). *Basic concepts and models for interpreter and translator training.* Philadelphia: Johns Benjamins.

Goldstein, B. (2000). *Cultural and linguistic diversity resource guide for speech-language pathologists.* San Diego, CA: Singular.

Gollnick, D.M., and Chinn, P.C. (1990). *Multicultural education in a pluralistic society.* Columbus, OH: Merrill.

Goodglass, H., and Kaplan, E. (1983). Boston Diagnostic Aphasia Examination. Philadelphia: Lean and Febiger.

Goodz, N.S. (1994). Interactions between parents and children. In F. Genessee (Ed.), *Educating second language children: The whole child, the whole curriculum, the whole community* (pp. 61–81). New York: Cambridge University Press.

Gopnick, A., and Choi, S. (1995). Names, relational words and cognitive development in English and Korean speakers. Nouns are not always learned before verbs. In M. Tomasello and W. Merriman (Eds.), *Beyond names for things: Young children's acquisition of verbs* (pp. 63–80). Hillsdale, NJ: Erlbaum.

Grimes, B.F. (Ed.). (1999). Top 100 languages by population. In *Ethnologue* [Electronic Version]. Retrieved June 1, 2001, from the World Wide Web: http://www.sil.org/ethnologue/top100.html

Gumpertz, J.J. (1982). *Discourse strategies.* New York: Cambridge University Press.

Gutiérrez-Clellen, V.F., Peña, E., and Quinn, R. (1995). Accounting cultural differences in narrative style: A multicultural perspective. *Topics in Language Disorders, 15*(4), 54–67.

Hall, E.T. (1976). *Beyond culture.* Garden City, NY: Anchor.

Hall, E.T. (1977). *The hidden dimension.* Garden City, NY: Anchor.

Hammer, C.S., and Weiss, A.L. (2000). African-American mothers views of their infants' language development and language learning environment. *American Journal of Speech-Language Pathology, 9*(2), 126–140.

Harding, E., and Riley, P. (1986). *The bilingual family: A handbook for parents.* New York: Cambridge University Press.

Harry, B. (1992). *Cultural diversity, families and the special education system.* New York: Teachers College Press.

Heath, S.B. (1983). *Ways with words.* New York: Cambridge University Press.

Hermes, D. (1998). Measuring perceptual similarity of pitch contours. *Journal of Speech and Hearing Research, 41,* 73–82.

Hiebert, E.H. (Ed.). (1991). *Literacy for a diverse society: Perspectives, practices and policies.* New York: Teachers College Press.

Hong, Y.Y., Morris, M.W, Chiu, C.Y., and Benet-Martínez, V. (2000). Multicultural minds: A dynamic constructivist approach to culture and cognition. *American Psychologist, 55*(7), 709–720.

Huarte, A., Molina, M., Manrique, M., Olleta, J., and García-Tapia, R. (1996). Protocolo para la valoración de la audición y el lenguaje, en lengua española, en un programa de implantes cocleares. *Acta Otorrinolaringológica Española, 47,* 1.

Huer, M.B. (1997). Culturally inclusive assessments for children using augmentative and alternative communication (AAC). *Journal of Children's Communication Development, 19*(1), 23–24.

Huer, M.B. (2000). Examining perceptions of graphic symbols across cultures: A preliminary study of the impact of culture/ethnicity. *Augmentative and Alternative Communication, 16*(3), 180–185.

Hughes, D., McGillivray, L., and Schmidek, M. (1997). *Guide to narrative language.* Eau Claire, WI: Thinking Publications.

Individuals with Disabilities Education Act (IDEA) Amendments, 20 U.S.C. § 1400 *et. seq.* (1997).

Kallen, J.L. (2000, May). *Bilingualism, disability, and self-expression: Wrongs and rights.* Presentation at the de Monfort Symposium, Trinity College, Dublin, Ireland.

Katzner, K. (1986). *The languages of the world.* London: Routledge.

Kayser, H. (1995). *Bilingual speech-language pathology: An Hispanic focus.* San Diego, CA: Singular.

Kayser, H. (1998). *Assessment and intervention resource for Hispanic children.* San Diego, CA: Singular.

Kiernan, B., and Swisher, L. (1990). The initial learning of novel English words: Two single-object experiments with minority-language children. *Journal of Speech and Hearing Research, 33,* 707–716.

Knapp, M.L. (1972). *Nonverbal communication in human interaction.* New York: Holt, Rinehart, and Winston.

Langdon, H.W. (1992a). Language communication and socio-cultural patterns in Hispanic families. In H.W. Langdon (with L.L. Cheng) (Ed.), *Hispanic children and adults with communication disorders: Assessment and intervention* (pp. 99–131). Gaithersburg, MD: Aspen.

Langdon, H.W. (1992b). Speech and language assessment of LEP/Bilingual Hispanic students. In H.W. Langdon with L.L. Cheng (Eds.), *Hispanic children and adults with communication disorders: Assessment and intervention.* (pp.201–271). Gaithersbug, MD: Aspen.

Langdon, H.W. (1999). Foreign accent: Implications for delivery of speech and language services. *Topics in Language Disorders, 19*(4), 49–64.

Langdon, H.W. (2002). *Interpreters and translators in communication disorders: A practitioner's handbook.* Eau Claire, WI: Thinking Publications.

Langdon, H.W. (in press). *Assessment of English learners with the collaboration of an interpreter/translator* [Video]. Rockville, MD: American Speech-Language-Hearing Association.

Langdon, H.W. (with L.L. Cheng) (Ed.). (1992) *Hispanic children and adults with communication disorders: Assessment and intervention.* Gaithersbug, MD: Aspen.

Langdon, H.W., and Clark, L. (1993). Profile of Hispanic/Latino American students. In E.W. Clark (Ed.), *Faculty and student challenges in facing cultural and linguistic diversity* (pp. 88–113). Springfield, IL: Thomas.

Langdon, H.W., and Merino, B. (1992). Acquisition and development of a second language in the Spanish-speaker. In H.W. Langdon (with L.L. Cheng) (Ed.), *Hispanic children and adults with communication disorders: Assessment and intervention* (pp. 132–167). Gaithersburg, MD: Aspen.

Langdon, H.W., and Saenz, T.I. (1996). *Language assessment and intervention with multicultural students: A guide for speech-language-hearing professionals.* Oceanside, CA: Academic Communication Associates.

Langdon, H.W., Siegel, V., Halog, L., and Sánchez-Boyce, M. (1994). *Interpreter translator manual in the educational setting.* Sacramento, CA: Resources in Special Education (RISE).

Leopold, W. (1970). *Speech development in a bilingual child* (Vol.1–4). New York: AMS Press.

Leung, B. (1995, March). *Non-biased assessment.* Workshop presented at Alliance 2000, Monterey, CA.

Lustig, M.W., and Koester, J. (1999). *Intercultural competence: Interpersonal communication across cultures.* New York: Longman.

Lynch, E., and Hanson, M. (1992). *Developing cross-cultural competence: A guide for working with young children.* Baltimore: Brookes.

Manuel-Dupont, S., and Yoakum, S. (1997). Training interpreter paraprofessionals to assist in the language assessment of English language learners in Utah. *Journal of Children's Communication Development, 18,*(1), 91–102.

Mares, S. (1980). Pruebas de Expresión Oral y Percepción de la Lengua Española (PEOPLE). Downey, CA: Los Angeles County Office of Education.

Martin-Jones, M. (1995). Code-switching in the classroom: Two decades of research. In L. Milroy and P. Muysken (Eds.), *One speaker, two languages* (pp. 90–110). New York: Cambridge University Press.

Matsuda, M., and O'Connor, L.C. (1993, April). *Creating an effective partnership: Training bilingual communication aides.* Paper presented at the California Speech-Language-Hearing Association Convention, Palm Springs, CA.

Mayer, M. and Mayer, M. (1975). *One frog too many.* New York: Dial Books.

McCullough, J., Wilson, R.H., Birck, J.D., and Anderson, L.G. (1994). A multimedia approach for estimating speech recognition of multilingual clients. *American Journal of Audiology, (3)*1, 19–24.

McGowan, R.J., Johnson, D.L., and Maxwell, S.E. (1981). Relations between infant behavior ratings and concurrent and subsequent mental test scores. *Developmental Psychology, 17*(5), 542–553.

McQuillan, J., and Tse, L. (1995). Child language brokering in linguistic minority communities: Effects on cultural inter-action, cognition, and literacy. *Language and Education, 9*(3), 195–213.

Menn, L., O'Connor, M., Obler, L.K., and Holland, A. (1995). *Non-fluent aphasia in a multilingual world.* Philadelphia: Johns Benjamins.

Meyerson, M.D. (1990). Cultural considerations in the treatment of Latinos with craniofacial malformations. *The Cleft Palate Journal, 27,* 279–288.

Michael, S. and Cocchini, J. (1997). Training college students as community interpreters: An innovative model. In S.E. Carr, R. Roberts, A. Dufour, and D. Steyn (Eds.), *The critical link: Interpreters in the community* (pp. 237–248). Philadelphia: Johns Benjamins.

Mikkelson, H., and Mintz, H. (1997). Orientation workshop for interpreters of all languages: How to strike a balance between the ideal world and reality. In S.E. Carr, R. Roberts, A. Dufour, and D. Steyn (Eds.), *The critical link: Interpreters in the community* (pp. 55–63). Philadelphia: Johns Benjamins.

Milroy, L., and Muysken, P. (Eds.). (1995). *One speaker, two languages.* New York: Cambridge University Press.

Mitchell, R., and Myles, F. (1998). *Second language learning theories.* London: Arnold.

Muñoz-Sandoval, A.F., Cummins, J., Alvarado, C.G., and Ruef, M. (1998). Bilingual Verbal Ability Tests (BVAT). Itasca, IL: Riverside.

Myers-Scotton, C. (1992). Comparing code-switching and borrowing. *Journal of Multilingual and Multicultural Development, 13*(1–2), 19–39.

Myers-Scotton, C. (1993). *Social motivation for codeswitching: Evidence from Africa.* Oxford: Clarendon Press.

National Clearinghouse for Bilingual Education. (1999) State K–12 LEP enrollment and top languages. Retrieved June 11, 2001, from the World Wide Web: http://www.ncbe.gwu.edu/ncbepubs/reports/state-data/index.htm

Nettle, D. (1999). _Linguistic diversity._ New York: Oxford University Press.

Nicholson, N.S., and Martinsen, B. (1997). Court interpretation in Denmark. In S.E. Carr, R. Roberts, A. Dufour, and D. Steyn (Eds.), _The critical link: Interpreters in the community_ (pp. 259–270). Philadelphia: Johns Benjamins.

Nicolosi, L., Harryman, E., and Krescheck, J. (1996). _Terminology of communication disorders: Speech-language-hearing_ (4th ed). Baltimore: Williams and Wilkans.

Nilsen, D.L.F., and Nilsen, A.P. (1973). _Pronunciation contrasts in English._ New York: Regents.

Ortíz, A.A., García, S.B., and Wilkinson, C.T. (1988, August). _Handicapped minority research institute: Five years in review._ General session presented at the Bilingual Special Education Summer Conference, Austin, Tx.

Pang, V.O., and Cheng, L.R. (1998). _Struggling to be heard: The unmet needs of the Asian Pacific American children._ Albany, NY: SUNY Press.

Parette, H.P., Brotherson, M.J., and Huer, M.B. (2000). Giving families a voice in augmentative and alternative communication decision making. _Education and Training in Mental Retardation and Developmental Disabilities, 35_(2), 177–190.

Pedersen, P., Draguns, J., Lonner, W., and Trimble, J. (1996). _Counseling across cultures._ Thousand Oaks, CA: Sage.

Penney, C., and Sammons, C. (1997). Training the community interpreter: The Nunavut Arctic college experience. In S.E. Carr, R. Roberts, A. Dufour, and D. Steyn (Eds.), _The critical link: Interpreters in the community_ (pp. 55–64). Philadelphia: Johns Benjamins.

Perozzi, J., and Sanchez, M. (1992). The effect of instruction in L1 on receptive acquisition of L2 for bilingual children with language delay. *Language, Speech, and Hearing Services in Schools, 23,* 348–352.

Pochhacker, F. (1997). "Is there anybody out there?" Community interpreting in Austria. In S.E. Carr, R. Roberts, A. Dufour, and D. Steyn (Eds.), *The critical link: Interpreters in the community* (pp. 215–226). Philadelphia: Johns Benjamins.

Poplack, S. (1980). Sometimes I'll start a sentence in Spanish Y TERMINO EN ESPANOL: Towards a typology of code-switching. *Linguistics, 18,* 581–618.

Puyuelo, S.M., Rondal, J.A., and Wiig, E.H. (2000). *Evaluación del lenguaje.* Barcelona, Spain: Masson.

Puyuelo, M., Wiig, E., Renom, J., and Solanas, A. (1998). Batería de Lenguaje Objectiva y Criterial (BLOC). Barcelona, Spain: Masson.

Registry of Interpreters for the Deaf. (2001). *Code of ethics.* Retrieved May 25, 2001 from the World Wide Web: http://www.rid.org/code.html

Reyes, B. (1995). Neurogenic communication disorders in bilingual adults. In H. Kayser (Ed.), *Bilingual speech-language pathology: An Hispanic focus* (pp. 153–182). San Diego, CA. Singular.

Roberts, R. (1997). Community interpreting today and tomorrow. In S.E. Carr, R. Roberts, A. DuFour and D. Steyn (Eds.), *The critical link: Interpreters in the community.* (pp.7–26). Philadelphia: Johns Benjamins.

Ronjat, J. (1913). _Le développement du langage observé chez un enfant bilingue._ Paris: Campion

Roseberry-McKibbin, C. (1995). _Multicultural students with special language needs: Practical strategies for assessment and intervention._ Oceanside, CA: Academic Communication Associates.

Roy, C.B. (2000). _Interpreting as a discourse process._ New York: Oxford University Press.

Ruhen, M. (1976). _A guide to languages of the world._ Stanford, CA: Stanford University Press.

Schinke-Llano, L. (1983). Foreigner talk in content classrooms. In H. Seliger and M. Long (Eds.), _Classroom oriented research in second language acquisition_ (pp. 146–168). Rowley, MA: Newbury.

Scollon, R., and Scollon, S.W. (1995). _Intercultural communication: A discourse approach._ Oxford, England: Blackwell.

Silliman, E.T., and Diehl, S.F. (1995). Foreword. _Topics in Language Disorders, 15_(4), vi–ix.

Skehan, P. (1988). Language testing. _Language Teaching, 21,_ 1–13; 211–222.

Smith, C.S. (2001, April 9). Collision with China: The semantics. _The Washington Post,_ p. 2B.

Strauss, R. (1990). Cultural considerations in the treatment of Latinos with craniofacial malformations. _Cleft Palate Journal, 27,_ 275–278.

Suárez-Orozco, M.M. (1989). _Central American refugees and U.S. high school: A psychological study and motivation._ Stanford, CA: Stanford University Press.

Tan, A. (1989). *The joy luck club.* New York: Putman.

Tharp, R.G., and Gallimore, R. (1991). *The instructional conversation: Teaching and learning in social activity.* Washington, DC: Center for Applied Linguistics.

Toliver-Weddington, G., and Meyerson, M.D. (1983). Training paraprofessionals for identification and intervention with the communicatively disordered bilingual. In D.R. Omark and J.G. Erickson (Eds.), *The bilingual exceptional child* (pp. 379–385). San Diego, CA: College Hill Press.

Trueba, H.T., Cheng, L.L., and Ima, K. (1993). *Myth or reality: Adaptive strategies of Asian Americans in California.* London: Falmer Press.

Trueba, H.T., Jacobs, L., and Kirton, E. (1990). *Cultural conflict and adaptation: The case of Hmong children in American society.* London: Falmer Press.

Tse, L. (1995). Language brokering among Latino adolescents: Prevalence, attitudes, and school performance. *Hispanic Journal of Behavioral Sciences, 17*(2), 180–193.

U.S. Bureau of the Census. (1990). Detailed language spoken at home and ability to speak english for persons 5 years and over—50 languages with greatest number of speakers: United States 1990. Retrieved May 25, 2001, from the World Wide Web: http://www.census.gov/population/socdemo/language/table5.txt

Valdés, G., and Figueroa, R.A. (1995). *Bilingualism and testing: A special case of bias.* Norwood, NJ: Ablex.

Valencia, R.R., and Rankin, R.J. (1985). Evidence of content bias on the MacArthur Scales with Mexican-American children:

Implications for test and nonbiased assessment. _Journal of Educational Psychology, 77_(2), 197–207.

van Kleeck, A. (1994). Potential bias in training parents as conversational partners with their children who have delays in language development. _American Journal of Speech-Language Pathology, 3_(1), 67–78.

Westby, C. (1990). Ethnographic interviewing: Asking the right questions to the right people in the right way. _Journal of Childhood Communication Disorders, 13,_ 101–111.

Westby, C., and Roman, R. (1995). Finding the balance: Learning to live in two worlds. _Topics in Language Disorders, 15_(4), 68–90.

Wiig, E., Secord, W., and Semel, E. (1997). Clinical Evaluation of Language Fundamentals–3 (CELF–3), Spanish Version. San Antonio, TX: Psychological Corporation.

Wilson, B. (1993). _Trouble in Transylvania: A Cassandra Reilly mystery._ Seattle, WA: Seal Press.

Wolfram, W., and Christian, D. (1989). _Dialects and education: Issues and answers._ Englewood Cliffs, NJ: Prentice Hall.

Wong-Fillmore, L. (1991). Second language learning in children: A model of language learning in social contexts. In E. Bialystok (Ed), _Language processing in bilingual children_ (pp. 49–69). New York: Cambridge University Press.

Woodcock, R.W. (1981). Woodcock Language Proficiency Battery: Spanish Version. Hingham, MA: Teaching Resources Corporation.

Zimmerman, I.L., Steiner, V.G., and Pond, R.E. (1993). Preschool Language Scale–3, Spanish Version. San Antonio, TX: Psychological Corporation.

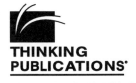